Praise for *Every Woman's Guide to Cycling*

"If you've ever thought about hopping on a bike to get in shape, this book is a must-have. Selene Yeager brings back the joy of cycling that you knew as a kid and provides you with the tools and know-how you need now to rediscover this form of exercise. Whether you're just starting out or you ride regularly, you'll be inspired by the stories of women just like you who've lost weight and gotten fit, and the simple training programs will help you reach your personal goals, too."

—Michele Stanten, Fitness Director, *Prevention* Magazine

EVERY WOMAN'S GUIDE TO
CYCLING

Everything You Need to Know,

from Buying Your First Bike

to Winning Your First Race

Selene Yeager

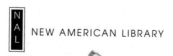

NEW AMERICAN LIBRARY

New American Library
Published by New American Library, a division of
Penguin Group (USA) Inc., 375 Hudson Street,
New York, New York 10014, USA
Penguin Group (Canada), 90 Eglinton Avenue East, Suite 700, Toronto,
Ontario M4P 2Y3, Canada (a division of Pearson Penguin Canada Inc.)
Penguin Books Ltd., 80 Strand, London WC2R 0RL, England
Penguin Ireland, 25 St. Stephen's Green, Dublin 2, Ireland
(a division of Penguin Books Ltd.)
Penguin Group (Australia), 250 Camberwell Road, Camberwell, Victoria 3124,
Australia (a division of Pearson Australia Group Pty. Ltd.)
Penguin Books India Pvt. Ltd., 11 Community Centre, Panchsheel Park,
New Delhi—110 017, India
Penguin Group (NZ), 67 Apollo Drive, Rosedale, North Shore 0632,
New Zealand (a division of Pearson New Zealand Ltd.)
Penguin Books (South Africa) (Pty.) Ltd., 24 Sturdee Avenue,
Rosebank, Johannesburg 2196, South Africa

Penguin Books Ltd., Registered Offices: 80 Strand, London WC2R 0RL, England

First published by New American Library, a division of Penguin Group (USA) Inc.

First Printing, March 2008

1 3 5 7 9 10 8 6 4 2

NAL
REGISTERED TRADEMARK—MARCA REGISTRADA
LIBRARY OF CONGRESS CATALOGING-IN-PUBLICATION DATA
Yeager, Selene.
Every woman's guide to cycling : everything you need to know, from buying your first bike
to winning your first race / Selene Yeager.
p. cm.
ISBN: 978-0-451-22304-3
1. Cycling.   2. Women cyclists.   I. Title.
GV1041.Y43 2008
796.6082—dc22   2007034251

Set in Berkeley
Designed by Patrice Sheridan

Printed in the United States of America

PUBLISHER'S NOTE
Outdoor recreational activities are by their very nature potentially hazardous. All participants in such activities must assume the responsibility for their own actions and safety.
If you have any health problems or medical conditions, consult with your physician before
undertaking any outdoor activities. The information contained in this guide book cannot
replace sound judgment and good decision making, which can help reduce risk exposure,
nor does the scope of this book allow for disclosure of all the potential hazards and risks
involved in such activities.
Learn as much as possible about the outdoor recreational activities in which you participate, prepare for the unexpected, and be cautious. The reward will be a safer and more
enjoyable experience.
The publisher does not have any control over and does not assume any responsibility
for author or third-party Web sites or their content.

Acknowledgments

No book is the product of one person. Without the support, assistance, and sometimes outright hand-holding of an amazing array of people, this book would not have come to life. I would like to thank my husband, Dave, my patron saint of patience; my daughter, Juniper, who though less patient is enormously understanding; my mom and dad for helping take care of life so I can work; my agent, Jeremy Katz, for making it happen; my editors, Claire Zion and Hilary Dowling, for sage wisdom and advice; James Herrera for brilliant programming and for overcoming insane obstacles to lend a helping hand; Liz Reap-Carlson for her indomitable spirit and skilled photography and editing; Steve Madden, Bill Strickland, and the rest of the *Bicycling* magazine staff who have taught me so much and always make me look good; and South Mountain Cycles and all the friends with whom I share so many miles and so much of my life. It's always a good ride.

Table of Contents

"Let me tell you what I think of bicycling. I think it has done more to emancipate women than anything else in the world. It gives women a feeling of freedom and self-reliance. I stand and rejoice every time I see a woman ride by on a wheel . . . the picture of free, untrammeled womanhood."

—SUSAN B. ANTHONY

1

Destination Cyclist

You Need to Ride!

When I was a young girl growing up in rural Pennsylvania, my first "adult" bike—a silver ten-speed Schwinn—was my personal ticket to paradise. I'd pull it out of the shed and off I went, away from the watchful eyes of my parents, away from all the pressures of high school BS, away to explore. I could dream and I could pretend—that I could fly, that I was someone else living in some other more exciting place. My bike represented unlimited potential. Anywhere my parents took me by car, I could get by my bike. On it was the only place I felt completely free.

Flash forward ten years. I was twenty-five, ten pounds overweight and coming out of a crappy job on the tail end of a bad mistake of a marriage. My bike, an okay Specialized hybrid, sat in the garage with a pair of flats. "Free" had fallen out of my vocabulary. Then I met some people who liked to ride bikes. They were much more "serious cyclists," but they invited me to join them. Grinning like an idiot, I rolled along quiet country roads, huffed and puffed my way up hills, and swooped and whooped down the other sides. My wings were back! And I used them to lift my life to a much better place.

In the dozen years that followed, my bike has taken me around the world, allowing me to enjoy the sights, sounds, and rich aromas of some of the most beautiful places on the globe in a way that is impossible off two wheels. I've used my bike to raise money to fight AIDS, cancer, and autism. I've tested my physical limits on some of the hardest racecourses our country has to offer. I've learned a lot about myself and have earned a few accolades along the way, not the least of which is being *Bicycling* magazine's Fit Chick and dishing out advice to fellow cycling enthusiasts each month. My bike has given me the freedom to realize my fullest potential. I guarantee it can do the same for you.

THE FREEDOM OF RIDING

The simple act of swinging your leg over a bike and pedaling away delivers nearly instant freedom. Start cycling now and you'll be free from:

ADULT DOLDRUMS

This is, hands down, the best part of riding. Feeling free from all the no-fun stuff of being an adult. The crushing responsibilities. The bills. The worries over the kids. The worries over aging parents. The worries over too many worries go out the window when you're on your bike. Nothing brings back that buried youthful exuberance like riding a bike. Nothing. Ride regularly, and you never have to feel like an overburdened adult again.

PRECONCEIVED NOTIONS

Too many women suffer from the "I could never . . ." syndrome. We have this idea of who we are all locked up, and we've locked up ourselves right along with it. The first time you get on a bike and ride forty, fifty, or even a hundred miles, you'll never say, "I could never" again.

BODY IMAGE TORTURE

Fat thighs, droopy butt, jiggly arms. Oh my, we women can torture ourselves. The best remedy for a bad body image is appreciation for what your body can do. It's very hard to hate a pair of legs that carry you to the top of a mountain. It's hard to feel bad about a body that gives you all the happiness of cycling. It's impossible to bellyache about your behind when you're glowing from a great ride. The women I ride with exude more physical confidence than all the dieting and plastic surgery in the world could ever provide.

WAISTLINE WOES

Okay. I'll fess up, it *is* easier to feel happier in your own skin when your skin isn't stretched over a couple more dress sizes than you'd like. Cycling not only makes you feel better about your body; it makes your body better too. It burns fat, lowers blood pressure, firms muscles, and all those things that make you look and feel great. Avid cyclists are known for their voracious appetites and low body fat. That's because even a moderate two-hour ride can easily kill off a thousand calories (that's about half a day's worth for many of us!). None of the women I ride with ever goes on a "diet." We use food for fuel—and, happily, we need a lot of fuel!

WOMEN ARE BUILT TO BIKE . . . AND NOW BIKES ARE BUILT FOR WOMEN

Women's bodies are built to ride a bike. We have naturally strong legs, perfectly suited for pedaling across rolling terrain. We're graced with endurance and steady fitness to go the extra mile—sometimes even when men can't. We're social. And few sports are more social than cycling. You can hear the laughter and rambling chitchat of a group of cyclists from a mile away. Finally, cycling is a gentle yet challenging sport that is easy on your joints, wonderful for your heart, sheds unwanted pounds and shapes a rear view you'll love. Anyone of any age or any fitness level can do it.

There's also never been a better time to be a woman in cycling. When I first started cycling seriously, I was one of only a handful of women on our regular local rides. Today when we roll out, the women often outnumber the men. Whereas the clothes used to be small men's stuff that was baggy and unflattering and not quite right anywhere, today's women-specific gear is fitted, fun, and full of flair. Some of the prettiest tops in my closet are made for cycling. Even bikes themselves come in women-specific designs, which offer more petite proportions for smaller riders.

Yet, despite all these emotional and physical benefits, many women remain hesitant to grab some wheels and go. Why? I believe it comes down to intimidation. They don't know what bike to buy. They're afraid of traffic. They're afraid of falling or having a sore butt. All legitimate concerns. And all easily overcome. All it takes is a little know-how (which you'll find in the pages to come) and the willingness to try. Don't believe me? Check out these women on wheels:

Kelly, an active thirty-something, had been taking my Spinning classes faithfully for years. Even on the sunniest May days when the fitness center echoed with emptiness, Kelly was there. Finally, after pedaling through enough make-believe rides to cross the country and back, Kelly showed up to class last year with a brand-new bike. She jumped into a few casual group rides to learn the rules of the road. One year later, she was doing some recreational racing at our local velodrome. "I'm already ready for a new, better bike!" she enthused last I saw her.

Or Joyce, an environmentally conscious politician in her forties who admired how confident and happy all the women she saw at her local bike shop looked. She wanted to feel that fit and vibrant as she got older and was elated that with a bike and a basket she could shed unwanted pounds, improve her energy, *and* reduce traffic and pollution on the roads around her home. A perfect trifecta! Today she's one of the biggest bike advocates I know.

Or Phyllis. Unhealthy and overweight in her early fifties, she decided to try indoor cycling as a gentle way to get in shape. My tales of

Saturday morning rides to the coffee shop, cycling vacations, and Century rides inspired her to take to the road. She too started by riding in small, casual groups to build her confidence. Nearly seventy dropped pounds later, my former student Phyllis is now a cycling instructor who specializes in leading rides for nervous newbies who want to experience the thrill of the sport. She's even begun racing and is kicking butt! She recently scored a gold medal at a state championship race and is now training to race on the national level. All because of a bike!

Still think you're too far gone to throw a leg over a bike? Talk to Jodya, who no doctor would believe was taking up cycling. She has diabetes. She's had a stroke. She smoked for the better part of forty-five years. She has neuropathy and a touch of emphysema. I could go on and on. As her trainer, I convinced her to put down the Benson & Hedges and pick up some dumbbells before her sixtieth birthday. As a cyclist, I inspired her to buy a mountain bike. She started riding the local canal path in her town. Before you knew it, she was riding twenty miles at a stretch. "Nothing feels as free as cycling," she once told me.

I believe all women should be free. That's why I wrote this book. I meet so many women who like the idea of riding, who would like to lose some weight and get in shape, who would maybe even love to try a triathlon (the women's market there is simply exploding), but they're unsure how to get rolling in the right direction. My goal is to provide straight-up, clear advice on everything you need to know: How to buy the right bike. What gear you really need, and what you don't. How to ride—really ride—your bike (climbing hills, riding fast, zipping through corners . . . it's all *so* much easier when you know the right techniques). How to train, maybe even race. How to eat to ride. How to fix simple stuff that can go wrong on the road. It's all here to set you on the road to cycling success.

HOW TO USE THIS GUIDE

When you're writing something for everybody, you run the risk of boring those already in the know and speaking over the heads of those just beginning. I would encourage new cyclists to start at the beginning of the book and read it in sequence. That way you'll learn all the lingo as you go along, and you won't be scratching your head when I refer to something in Chapter 7 that I defined in detail in Chapter 4.

Cyclists with a few miles under their tires can do a little more skipping around, but I would suggest at least skimming all the chapters. You're actually in the position to learn the most because you have a solid point of reference given your riding experience. For instance, you might be tempted to skip a chapter on "How to Ride"—I mean, you know how to ride if you've been riding, right? Sure, but when you're talking about skills such as cornering and climbing, you have to do them a few times to really get the feeling of how the bike works and reacts. Then when you read specific tips and techniques, they're more likely to click, and you'll be better able to try them next time you're out on the road. The same goes for chapters on gearing up and buying a bike. Even the most experienced cyclist can always pick up pointers that will help them find just what they need.

My hope is that this book will serve as a reference you can tap into throughout your cycling career. That you'll keep learning as you go and feel clear and confident from your maiden voyage to your first trip across a finish line.

Now turn the page and let's roll.

2

Finding the Right Ride

*How to Find Your Dream
Bike . . . Whatever
Your Dreams*

Most new cyclists come into the sport wanting "a bike"—
meaning a machine that rolls on two wheels when you
pedal it. They don't realize that, like cars, boats, and even
screwdrivers, each bike is designed to perform a very specific job.
And there are *a lot* to choose from. Taking a few moments to consider
what you want to do on your new bike (and what you want your new
bike to do) will prevent you from careening down a path littered with
good intentions, bad decisions, frustration, and buyer's remorse. I
know. I've worn a smooth groove down that road.

When I got back into riding, I did what millions of well-
intentioned women do every year: I walked into my local bike shop
and said, "I want a bike." To the salesman's credit, he did ask me a few
questions about what kind of riding I planned to do. But regrettably, I
hadn't given it much thought. I had finally gotten up the cash (and the
nerve) to invest in a good ride, and I didn't want to be bothered with
a game of twenty questions. I just wanted a bike. So, I mumbled
something about local trails and riding around the neighborhood and
ended up shelling out $700 (not a shabby chunk of change at the
time) for a ho-hum, half-decent hybrid (a half road, half off-road bike)

that I ditched six months later for a real road bike. Despite being al-most twenty years wiser, I recently blew it again when buying a new mountain bike (adjusting for inflation, the mistake was equally costly). I bought a bike that was more comfortable than zippy. I was wooed by marketing hype rather than sold on something that would fit my rid-ing style and wants (above all, I like to go fast) because I didn't follow my own very fundamental rule: *Know why you want to ride.*

LOOK DOWN THE ROAD

First ask yourself, "What's enticing me toward cycling?" Does your local Spinning class leave you longing for a taste of the real thing? Did a girlfriend just finish her first triathlon and is in the greatest shape (and happiest place) of her life? Do you want to start riding to work to get in shape and help fight global warming? Did you dabble in moun-tain biking on a vacation and now are hooked? Are some extra pounds dragging you down and you're hunting for some exercise that doesn't feel like a chore? Are you just looking for a fun way to get some fresh air and stress relief? Knowing what is bringing you to the sport is key to getting maximum enjoyment out of it.

Once you've answered the here and now questions, look down the road and try to project how you'll be riding in the near and fur-ther out future. Ideally, you'd like to buy a bike that you'll be happy with for at least three years. Will you be satisfied sticking to the local park trails? Or do you think you'd like to try more challenging moun-tain biking? Is there a local cycling group you'd like to join? Is a tri-athlon in your future? Does tackling a charity ride sound like fun? Would you like to do a bike tour of Vermont or Colorado someday?

If you're upgrading to a high-end ride, you might want it to last five or ten years, maybe be a companion for life. Gaze into that crystal ball inside your mind and see where you'd like the sport of cycling to take you. Sure, you may surprise yourself (none of us can really see the future), shed thirty pounds, ride across the country, and start a second career as a recreational racer as did my friend Phyllis. But the clearer a picture you can get now, the easier it will be to buy the right bike and get rolling in the right direction.

"BUT I ALREADY HAVE A BIKE"

Maybe you're thinking, "I can skip this chapter. I already have a bike." If all you need to do to get started is dust off your old bike and pump up the tires, that's great. But if your bike is more than ten years old and has been collecting dust and rust for years, a new bike might be in order, especially if the one you have came from a department store or was a hand-me-down. Bike technology has exploded during the past decade, and today's bikes are lighter, perform better, and are a whole lot more fun to ride than their predecessors.

What's more, that old bike may not be suited to carry you to your new goals. While almost any bike is fine for bumming around town or tooling around your local park with your kids, if you want to ride any kind of distance or take it out on the open road, riding a heavy cruiser or old mountain bike may end up feeling more like work than invigorating exercise.

So, even if you have a bike buried in your garage, go ahead and take the self-assessments in this chapter. Learn about your options and make sure it's the right ride for you. If you find out it is, fabulous! Just be sure to take it to your local shop for a tune-up before you go any distance on it. Time and disuse can take a toll on a bike's key components (like brakes and shifters). Your local bike mechanic can tighten up all the nuts and bolts, lube the moving parts, and make sure you're ready to roll safely.

CHOICES GALORE!

Shopping for a bike is a little bit like dating: There's a lot to choose from and you need to try a few out before making a commitment. As with mates, the best one may be the one you never dreamed of considering. By now, you should have at least a general idea of the type of bike you want—road or off-road. Here is a look at the bikes you'll be choosing from and what makes them specially suited to the jobs they do.

ROAD

In a nutshell

Built for speed. When you saw Lance Armstrong dancing on the pedals in the Tour de France, it was on a road bike.

Special features

The frame is made of lightweight materials like aluminum, high-quality steel, titanium, or in the case of very high-end bikes, carbon fiber (you'll find more on materials below). Curved "drop" handlebars allow you to tuck into a fast, aerodynamic position. The tires are skinny for the least amount of rolling resistance on the road.

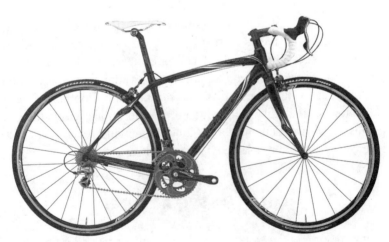

Enthusiast: With their slim, light frames and aerodynamically dropped handlebars, road bikes are built to slice through the air effortlessly.
Photo courtesy Specialized Bicycle Components.

Variations on the theme

- **Racing:** At the top of this category are the racers, where every detail from the number of spokes to the shape of the saddle (seat) is designed for minimum weight, maximum aerodynamics, and top speed. These are literally dream machines. But depending on your skill and interest level, some models in this category may be more bike than you need . . . or want. High-speed race machines aren't necessarily built for comfort. In fact, they can be pretty "stiff" (meaning the frame doesn't have much flex or give), which can leave you feeling beat up on long rides, especially over rough roads. Top-level racing bikes are often also "twitchy." They're built to be ultra-responsive to react to every flick of a pro rider's wrist. Less experienced riders may not like the "nervous" feeling of a bike that seems to over-respond to every little movement. That said, there are plenty of race-worthy bikes that are comfy enough to ride all day. If you're buying in this category, test-drive a few to find one that feels fast yet safely maneuverable. Bikes in this category generally cost $4,000 and more.
- **Enthusiast:** Most serious cyclists eventually end up buying a bike in this category. These bikes are race ready but also super fun. They're light and maneuverable yet stable and durable. You can climb like a rocket, descend like a missile, and speed along straightaways. Bicycles for the enthusiast come equipped with some of the highest quality components, so shifting and braking are buttery and smooth. Expect to pay $2,000 to $4,000 for bikes in this category.
- **Recreational:** Built to be quick and nimble, these bikes are no slouches, but they often are designed with a greater eye toward comfort and stability than their race-specific brethren, so even a novice feels confident and at ease during long rides. For many, this is a great first bike of choice. It's forgiving enough to learn basic bike handling skills like quick cornering, comfy enough to ride your first century (100-mile

ride), but also efficient enough to let you hang with faster friends. Expect to pay $700 to $2,000 for a high-quality recreational bike. Lower priced recreational bikes are perfect for fitness riding and having fun, but they tend to be heavier with less smooth performance than bikes that cost a couple hundred dollars more.

- **Touring:** Built for comfort, touring bikes are like fine workhorses. They hold a lot of stuff, take a lot of abuse, and keep coming back for more. The riding position is more upright than aerodynamic, though the handlebars are still curved, so all-day riding is never a pain in the neck. Touring bikes also tend to be heavier and come equipped with fatter tires and mounts for racks and packs. They are best suited to riders who plan to load up and go somewhere. Cost varies widely, with quality bikes ranging from $700 to as much as $3,000.

- **Triathlon/Time Trial:** Designed to slice through the air at top speed, tri and time trial (TT) bikes (they are very similar) are all about aerodynamics. They come equipped with aerobars, bullhorn-shaped bars that stretch you low over the bike, so you can completely tuck down and slice through the wind, and they sometimes have smaller wheels. If your ultimate goal is to train for and compete in a triathlon, a tri bike is a good investment. Otherwise, consider buying a quality road bike and clip-on aerobars instead. Triathlon-specific bikes are not designed for long-ride comfort, and classic aerobars can be dangerous on regular road rides because the brakes and shifters are far removed from each other and the handling is twitchy. They're designed to go really fast in a straight line with no one around you. Some charity rides forbid bikes with aerobars because they're not safe in group riding conditions. Expect to pay $1,500 and more for a quality TT bike.

How it fits and feels

To the noncycling bystander, road bikes look rather uncomfortable with their narrow seats, skinny tires, and low, curvy handlebars. If you haven't ridden in a while, the first time out may feel a little awkward. But a proper-fitting road bike should feel comfortable from the get-go, as if you're part of the machine. Your weight should feel evenly positioned between your butt, your hands, and your feet. You should feel balanced, not too stretched out or too scrunched up. You'll spend the majority of your riding time with your hands on the brake hoods (the curved top parts of the brakes that extend from the bars), but you should be able to reach and pedal comfortably with your hands down in the lowest position of the "drops" (the bottom of the bars) as well.

Important considerations

One overlooked yet very important road bike feature that will profoundly impact how much you enjoy your new ride is your gears. As you'll learn later on, your goal should be to be able to pedal comfortably whether the road resembles a pancake or a party hat. That means having plenty of gears to choose from, especially those on the easier end of the spectrum. Most road bikes come with either a nine- or ten-speed cassette. That means there are nine or ten gears on the rear wheel. Up front, there are either two or three chainrings (the gears the chain sits on by the pedals). If there are three chainrings in the front and ten gears in the back, you have a whole lot of gears to choose from, but you also have a little more weight from the extra chainring and a little more hassle navigating all those gear combinations.

If you're already pretty fit and fast or ride mostly on flat terrain, you're fine to go with a standard double chainring setup. If you live in the mountains or you're just getting into riding and plan on hitting some serious hills, a triple chainring is likely the way to go. One other alternative: a *compact* double chainring setup. Compact chainrings are smaller than a standard double, so the gearing skews easier without having an added chainring. Talk to the salesperson at your bike shop about the type of riding you plan to do as well as your fitness level and any orthopedic issues you may have (for example, people with bad knees may prefer low climbing gears).

MOUNTAIN

In a nutshell

Off-road fun. Built to ride over rocks, roots, and bumpy terrain without bucking you off.

Special features

Fat, knobby tires provide excellent traction on sketchy surfaces. Straight, wide handlebars give you leverage to pull the front tire over obstacles and provide better steering control. The handlebars are higher so you're in a more upright riding position, which lets you manipulate the bike more easily. The top tube (the bar that sits between your legs) slopes down at a steep angle, providing ample clearance between your body and the bike, so you don't ram your girl parts into the frame if you have to jump off quickly.

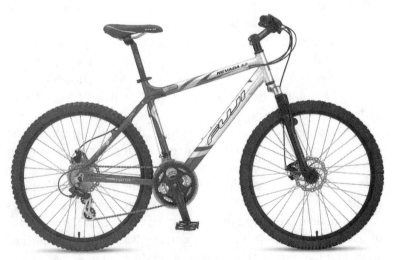

Hardtail: Mountain bikes have front-end suspension and disc brakes to help with rough riding on trails.
Photo courtesy of Fuji Bicycles

Variations on the theme

- **_Hardtail:_** Mountain bikes are largely defined by their suspension or shock absorbers. Bikes made for relatively smooth terrain like cinder paths or hard-packed dirt trails need a whole lot less shock absorption to keep you rolling along comfortably than bikes made to bomb down rock- and log-strewn wooded paths. Hardtails are so called because though they have a shock absorber for the front wheel (nearly all mountain bikes do), they have none in the rear. The advantage of hardtails is they tend to be zippier, since the back end is lighter and the power from your pedals goes right into propelling you forward without getting absorbed by the rear shock. They also tend to be considerably less expensive. The downside is that your butt becomes the shock absorber on rough terrain, and it can be more challenging to keep traction (a rear shock helps keep your rear wheel from bouncing all over the place). If you have no plans to tackle challenging terrain, you'll be perfectly happy with a hardtail. Prices range from $300 to $800.

- **_Cross-country Suspension:_** These bikes are designed to eat up the bumps on the trail without slowing you down. They generally have light rear suspension that allows the bike to absorb rocks and roots while keeping the back tire down. These bikes are built for speed, not necessarily all-day comfort or serious shock absorption. They're perfect if you like to go fast (maybe even race) and don't expect a cushy ride over rough terrain. Expect to pay anywhere from $900 to $5,000. Many great bikes come in at around $1,500.

- **_All-Mountain:_** The bombers of the bunch. As the name implies, these bikes are made to take whatever the mountain has to offer. If you're a dirt girl at heart and long to tackle challenging terrain with a bike built to take the abuse, an all-mountain ride may be the way to go. They have more beefy rear suspension systems that can absorb bigger hits without bucking you off. They're generally not quite as zippy as cross-country mountain bikes (though they're still fast), but they're more plush so you can spend long days in the saddle without an aching behind. They are similarly priced to cross-country suspension bikes.

How it fits and feels

In a word, comfy. Because you sit upright (like on your old banana-seat bike you had as a kid), mountain bikes feel very natural from the get-go. They're also lower to the ground and more compact than road bikes, so you should feel very stable. Out on the trail is the real test. You obviously need some special skills to ride technical (challenging) terrain, but a good mountain bike should feel very easy to maneuver. Because they have big tires with lots of knobs on them, mountain bikes feel a little slow and ungainly on pavement. If you want a very cushy bike, but aren't looking to go off-road, check out a hybrid (see below); don't buy a mountain bike.

Important considerations

Components! Pay close attention to brakes and shifting systems, which take a beating in typical off-road riding conditions. Higher-end mountain bikes come with what are known as disc brakes. Unlike traditional brakes that squeeze the rim of your wheel to slow you down, disc brakes work by squeezing a metal plate that is attached at the center of the wheel. They're heavier and more complex to fix should something go wrong, but they work infinitely better in muddy, wet, gritty conditions, where rim brakes often fail. If you intend to ride in all weather and on all terrain, they're worth the added cost. Ditto for shifting systems. Inexpensive mountain bikes usually come with low-end shifting systems that work okay in dry, nonstressful riding situations but not as well in demanding conditions. Clean, crisp, reliable shifting increases the pleasure of a mountain bike ride exponentially (as opposed to having your chain jumping around on the gears or not moving when you want to shift). Again, if you're serious about getting into off-road riding, it's worth paying a little extra up front for quality components that are built to perform under pressure.

HYBRID

In a nutshell

A little bit road, a little bit off-road. Does neither spectacularly but both reasonably well.

Special features

Medium-size tires let you roll briskly yet provide stability on moderately bumpy terrain like rough roads and cinder paths. The head-up, traffic-friendly position provides added comfort and lets you peer easily down the road, making hybrids good commuting and all-around exercise bikes.

Variations on the theme

- **Flat-bar Road:** The low, curvy handlebars of traditional road bikes are a turnoff for some riders. So bike manufacturers invented the flat-bar road bike. These bikes are built to provide road speed with mountain bike comfort. The downside of the flat bar: limited hand positions. There are three or four different places to rest your hands on a curved bar, giving your upper body a break from being in the same position mile after mile. If you go with a flat bar, look for one with bar ends, extensions at the end of the handlebars that allow another option for gripping the bar. Expect to spend anywhere from $450 to $1,200, depending on the quality of materials and components.
- **Cyclocross:** The SUV of road bikes, cross bikes were developed for winter dirt track races that involve riding around an off-road loop and jumping off and running the bike over various obstacles. They're generally made of lightweight

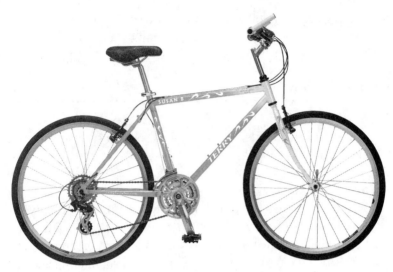

Flat-bar road bike: Hybrids blend the shock-absorption of a mountain bike with some of the aerodynamics of a road bike frame for a comfortable all-around ride.
Ron Wu Photo

materials and have beefy (but not fat) tires. Because they're designed to stay upright in sketchy conditions, cross bikes offer great handling and stability as well as durability. They can be a good choice for a rider who doesn't need the fastest bike on the road and who also is interested in some mild off-road riding. Like SUVs, cross bikes don't come cheap, however. Costs hover in the $1,100 to $2,500 range.

How it fits and feels

Hybrids fit similar to road bikes but generally put your body in a less aggressive position. They ride similarly well on pavement and on dirt. Again, they don't cruise along the pavement as buttery as a road bike and they won't stand up to very many rocks or roots off road, but these Jills-of-all-trades are lovely in the gray areas in between.

Important considerations

Buyer's remorse. You should make the decision to buy a hybrid, not buy one out of indecision. If your goal is charity rides and long weekend spins in the country, don't buy a hybrid just in case you want to try off-road riding. Buy a hybrid if you know you want a bike that will do a little bit of everything well enough.

URBAN/COMMUTER

In a nutshell

Need to hit the bank and the post office, and grab a cup of cappuccino? A city bike is the ticket.

Special features

Relaxed, upright position allows you to sit comfortably while wearing a backpack or messenger bag slung over your shoulder. Wider tires are built to breeze over bumps and potholes. Many have fenders to keep your work clothes clean and may have racks for extra cargo.

Variations on the theme

- **Commuter:** These are strictly utilitarian machines built to buzz around town and carry you and your stuff from point to point. Some models come equipped with lights that are powered on when you pedal. Expect to pay $350 to $900.
- **Cruiser:** Stop by any family bike shop and you'll see colorful, sexy beach-style cruisers lined up on the pavement. These bikes have wide seats and handlebars that allow you to sit straight up and eat an ice cream cone or sip a latte while pedaling down the boardwalk. Expect to pay $250 to $550.

How it fits and feels

Similar to a hybrid, but often even more upright. A line of city bikes called Townies, made by Electra, actually lets you put your feet flat on the ground while you're firmly planted on the seat. These bikes

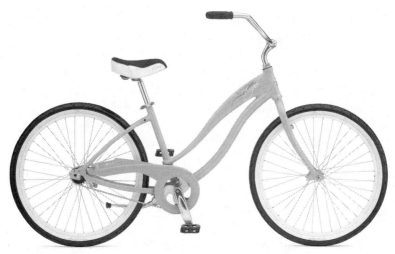

Cruiser: With their cushy seats and upright sitting position, cruisers are built for comfortable and relaxed riding.
Photo courtesy of Topeak

are built to feel sturdy. Their goal is to get you from here to there in comfort and style. They're not built for speed. Though they may feel comfortable for banging around town, you wouldn't want to ride forty miles on one. It would simply take too long.

Important considerations

Not many. These bikes are a low-risk investment. Even if you decide you love riding so much that you want to get into the sport more seriously, you can hang on to this workhorse for your everyday city needs, while you search for a more serious steed for longer adventures.

YOU GET WHAT YOU PAY FOR

Unless you're *really* well versed in bike manufacturing, it's hard to look at a $3,000 bike and not scratch your head and say, "What the hell makes it cost so much?" Rest assured, paying a couple thousand dollars for a bike isn't the same as shelling out $300 for designer jeans. You're buying craftsmanship and quality materials, not just a brand. Here's a breakdown of where the money goes:

FRAME

The bike frame is the body of the bike sans anything else: And I mean *anything* else—handlebars, wheels, gears, brakes, even the fork (the part that connects the handlebars to the front wheel; see below) are all separate entities. The material the frame is made from profoundly affects performance and ride quality. You can choose from:

Carbon fiber

Space-agey. This is a composite material made of tightly woven and hardened thin strands of carbon. It is all the rage in the aerospace industry and high-end road bikes. It's ultra-light and very responsive yet absorbs some of the road chatter, for a smooth ride. It's also pricey, so a whole bike made of the stuff doesn't come cheap. You can find some less expensive frames that use bits of carbon in the fork, handlebars, or other parts of the frame to lighten the weight and improve the ride quality. It's important to note that while carbon fiber is strong and durable, if you have a crash, you may have to kiss the frame good-bye. Carbon fiber can fail fast (an obviously very dangerous situation) once it's cracked. Many manufacturers have carbon fiber crash replacement policies.

Aluminum

Light, stiff, and fast. Aluminum frames are snappy and responsive—great if you love racy performance, which is why many race bikes are made from this material. Because it's relatively inexpensive, many entry-level and recreational- and enthusiast-level road bikes are made of aluminum. The downside to light, responsive aluminum is that it also can be bone-chatteringly stiff. For a softer ride, look for a bike that comes equipped with carbon fiber seat stays (the tubes that connect the back tire to your seat post area) and/or fork.

Titanium

Back in the '90s, titanium was the frame material du jour for top-of-the-line rides. Carbon fiber has tossed it from the throne, but there are still some mighty nice ti bikes, and they still don't come cheap. Aside from being light and responsive, titanium is almost literally bombproof. (I once saw a titanium Litespeed fly off a car going 70 MPH and cartwheel like a metallic tumbleweed down the Pennsylvania interstate without enduring a single ding. My friend rode it the same day.)

Steel/Chromoly

Traditional steel frames are still popular, especially for touring bikes, which need to be strong and durable during everyday wear, tear, and banging around. Steel is often the material of choice for entry-level bikes, but that doesn't mean all steel is inexpensive. High-quality Reynolds steel can carry the same price tag as other materials. The one downside of steel is the potential for rust.

FORK

This is the tuning fork–shaped component that attaches the front wheel to the frame and handlebars. (You'd expect it to be part of the frame, but it's a separate part.) Quality forks earn their higher price tag by sucking up road vibration and providing a smoother ride. Most road riders don't think about their forks too much, but a fork can make or break a ride off-road. Mountain bikes come with suspension forks that are quite literally shock absorbers. Their job is to cushion big blows and keep your front tire down (and your shoulders from taking a beating) over bumpy terrain. A high-end suspension fork can cost nearly as much as the bike itself.

COMPONENTS

These are the parts that literally make your bike go . . . and stop. Don't shrug these off; they are nearly as important as, if not more important than, your frame for determining the quality of your ride. If your bike rolls like silk, shifts crisply, and brakes smoothly, you're in for a dreamy ride. A bike that won't shift or come to a smooth stop, on the other hand, can be just short of a nightmare. Don't just tool around the parking lot on your test ride. Take the bike around the block and shift through all your gears. Come to a few quick stops. Does the bike respond quickly? It should.

Wheels

High-quality wheels blend light weight with stability and strength. As the price drops, the weight generally rises. This is important because heavier wheels take more energy to get rolling and keep rolling, so the ride is a little more difficult. But truth be told, unless the wheels are really cheap, you probably won't notice much difference from bike to bike.

Shifters/Derailleurs

Many bikes come with twenty speeds (more on a triple chainring). The shifters (which are on the handlebars) and the derailleurs (chain guides near the front chainrings and back gears) guide your chain from gear to gear. There are a number of shifting systems (Shimano, SRAM, and Campagnolo are popular makes). What's most important is they work smoothly (off-road, you'll also want durability, since they'll take more punishment). Top-of-the-line shifters and derailleurs move the chain easily and reliably and don't add much weight to the bike.

Brakes

Road bikes generally have rim brakes, which simply means that two pads squeeze the rim to slow you down when you apply the brakes. Mountain bikes, as mentioned above, come with either rim brakes or disc brakes. Disc brakes are more expensive, but they out-perform rim brakes in mucky conditions.

Pedals

This may come as a surprise, but the more you pay for a road bike the less likely it is to come with pedals (mountain bikes gener-ally do). Why's that? Because most cyclists ride what are called clip-less pedals, which is a small pedal platform that literally attaches to a cleat on your shoe. There are lots of pedal systems to choose from and everyone has their preference, so the manufacturers don't in-clude them. Of course, if you don't have a bike, you don't have ped-als, so you'll need to buy some. The shop can help you pick a pedal that best suits you or may even throw in a cheap pair to get you going until you decide.

WHAT BIKE SHOULD I BUY?

This is the million-dollar question. When faced with a dizzying array of choices, how do you know what's right for you? The ultimate goal is to match the kind of ride the bike provides with the kind you want to do. Since I know firsthand that can be a whole lot easier said than done, I've created this basic bike finder. Answer the following ques-tions about your riding style, bike dreams, personality traits, and lifestyle to help determine which bike type is best for you.

PART I: WHERE WILL YOU RIDE?

Questions:
1) I want to ride mostly on . . .
   A. Roads in my surrounding area
   B. Cinder paths, parks, rail-to-trail systems, around town
   C. Off-road, mountain bike trails, rough terrain

2) I expect my bike to . . .
  A. Do one thing (e.g., handle off-road challenges like rocks and roots or roll smoothly on the pavement) and do it well.
  B. Be a jack-of-all-trades. I don't know enough about what kind of riding I like to fully commit.
  C. Be suited for one kind of riding but offer some flexibility in case I want to try something a little different.

Answers:
1) *Your answer to Question 1 makes the big bike choice easy. If you chose:*
  A. You need a road bike.
  B. You need one of the many comfort/hybrid/commuter bikes available.
  C. You need a mountain bike.

2) *Your answer to Question 2 will help you narrow down your selection from Question 1. If you chose:*
  A. You want a purebred bike that is designed for your singular riding needs. Anything else will fall short.
  B. Consider a quality hybrid design. You can buy a flat-bar road bike or a cyclocross bike. You can also consider a hardtail mountain bike with minimal suspension that can handle small bumps but won't be cumbersome and slow on the pavement, or a commuting bike.
  C. Same as above. For the best bike, try to be as honest as possible with yourself. Maybe you like the idea of off-road riding, but if there are no trails nearby, the reality is you won't likely do it very often. Determine where you see yourself riding most and choose a bike that leans most heavily in that direction.

PART II: HOW WILL YOU RIDE?

Questions:

1) I want my bike to be . . .
   A. Race ready. I plan on riding with a serious group and maybe even compete.
   B. Comfortable and reliable. I'd like to take it out mostly on weekends for fresh air, exercise, and riding around town. I don't want a clunker, but I don't need top performance.
   C. Fast, fun, and durable. I'm a weekend warrior, so I want my bike to stand up to some abuse and still give solid performance.

2) Down the road, I see myself . . .
   A. Staying just as I am. I don't anticipate changing my riding style in the next two or three years.
   B. Improving. I'm a novice now, but I hope to learn and grow enough to take on some simple challenges like longer charity rides or short triathlons.
   C. As a serious cyclist, baby. I want to fly up hills and tackle challenging rides.

Answers:

1) *Within each bike category there are various price points that determine the quality of ride you will receive. Your answer to Question 1 helps define your price point. If you chose:*
   A. Splurge now. High-end bikes run in the $4,000-and-more range (yep, you read that right). But if you want top performance, it's *well* worth it. Like any investment, it'll sting a little at the initial impact, but you will be far happier down the road. A bike at this price is unbelievably beautiful on every level and will last a lifetime. If you just can't shell out that kind of change, go high-end enthusiast.

B. Entry level is the way to go. If you don't have great expectations, a no-frills ride around $500 to $700 will do you just fine. Don't go bargain basement, however. You still want a bike that runs smoothly and you can count on to brake and shift smoothly.

C. Go recreational to enthusiast. Right now is a great time to buy a bike in this category. For in the neighborhood of $900 to $2,000, you can get a whole lot of bike—one that will carry you from dabbling newbie to serious cyclist and beyond. For $2,000 to $4,000, you'll get a dreamy machine you'll love for years.

2) *Don't make the classic mistake of buying a bike today that you will regret tomorrow. If you're reading this book, chances are you plan on making cycling your new sport. Your answer to Question 2 helps ensure you buy a bike that will grow with you. Remember, you want to be happy on this bike for at least three years, longer if you're upgrading. If you chose:*

A. Fair enough. Invest in a quality bike in the right category and price point and ride to your heart's content.

B. Buy at the top end of your price point. Consider entering the next price point if you have any suspicion that you'll be looking to upgrade within three years.

C. Don't sell yourself short. What's "good enough" now will leave you longing for more in a season (or less). You don't have to take out a second mortgage or buy a pro-level ride, but you should consider going directly to the high-end recreational or enthusiast category for your first bike.

PART III: THE HUMAN MACHINE

Questions:

1) My physical condition is . . .
   A. Great. I may have a few excess pounds, but I'm generally healthy, fit, and reasonably flexible.
   B. So-so. I've got more than a few extra pounds and general aches and pains.
   C. Uh . . . let's not talk about that. (In truth, there are some serious limitations.)

2) When it comes to riding a bike, I'm . . .
   A. Green as a spring meadow. I haven't really ridden a bike since I could drive a car, and I've never been the most athletic woman on the planet. Truth be told, I'm kind of clumsy.
   B. Fairly skilled. I've ridden enough during my adulthood to feel comfortable climbing on a bike and pedaling away. And even if I haven't, I've stayed pretty active in other physical activities, so I won't be too rusty after a ride or two.
   C. Experienced. I would consider myself athletic, and I feel confident in my ability.

Answers:

1) *Generally speaking, how fit or unfit you are shouldn't impact the bike you buy. However, it's no big secret that the bent-over biking position can be a challenge for people who are very inflexible, have existing back pain, or have other orthopedic issues. If you chose:*
   A. Any bike (in your size, of course) will fit you just fine.
   B. You'll likely be okay with any bike you buy. If you have a history of back or neck issues, let the shop know and they'll steer you toward a bike that allows a slightly more

relaxed and/or upright position (i.e., there's only a small, if any, drop between the seat and handlebar height).

C.   There's a saying in the cycling industry: If you can't walk, crawl, or hobble, you can still ride a bike. In fact, many people who have pain during other activities roll along in complete comfort. However, be up front about any physical limitations when you're buying your bike. If you have limited mobility due to herniated discs, replaced hips, or excess weight, the salesperson can put you on a bike that will offer comfort in your range of motion.

2)   *Like cars, every bike offers a different type of ride. Some are highly responsive (not always the best quality for newbies); others respond only to a more firm touch. Question 2 will help steer you in the right direction. If you answered:*

A.   There's no shame in being a little physically awkward. The important thing is admitting it. You don't need training wheels, but no matter how fit you are, you should look for a bike that forgives rider error. Tell your bike shop you don't want anything too "nervous" or "twitchy," as some high-end bikes can be.

B.   You can sacrifice some stability for performance. If you don't have orthopedic issues that require a more relaxed ride, experiment with some more aggressive bike setups and see what feels best.

C.   If you're athletic with no physical limitations, err toward a setup designed for speed and quick handling.

PART IV: WHO I AM

Questions:

1)   When I make a purchase, I want . . .

A.   The best. I like plasma, high-def TVs, Lexuses, and stainless-steel appliances.

    B. Value. I don't mind spending a little more for the digital camera with more megapixels, but there's a diminishing point of returns. I don't need pro-level gear.

    C. Function. I expect what I buy—my Dell, my MP3 player, my TV—to work, but I don't ask a whole lot of it.

2) When I start a new hobby or interest, I typically stick with it like . . .

    A. Gum under a desktop. I'm in it for the ages.

    B. Suction cups. Some stick. Some plummet to the floor. The garage is littered with unused skis, golf clubs, and other equipment.

    C. A celebrity marriage. I love it to death for a few years, then move along to the next thing.

Answers:

1) *I ask these questions because many women (and men) who are new to the sport don't put bicycles in the same category as other major purchases. Maybe it's the "toy" reputation of the bicycle, or the fact that the prospective buyers haven't ever bought a bike for themselves (many people have only the bikes they received as presents as kids or teens), but people neglect to recognize the bicycle as a serious piece of machinery. Your answer to Question 1 will help you put your investment in perspective. If you chose:*

    A. Consider your new bicycle as being in the same category as a new car or TV. You really do get what you pay for (to a point . . . you can spend $10,000 on a bike if you *really* want to, but truly jaw-dropping bikes come in at around $5K), so go for a high-quality bike in your category.

    B. When buying a bike, being willing to spend a couple hundred bucks more often means the difference between a good bike and a really, really great bike. Keep that in mind if a salesperson steers you toward something slightly out of your price range but that he or she believes is a better deal. Most bike shop employees are very honest and won't try to sell you more than they think you need (often quite the opposite actually!).

C. You can get a very functional bike for about $500 to $700, but spend less and you run the risk of little annoyances like bad shifting, sloppy braking, and general heaviness putting a big damper on your ride. Light, well-performing bikes are simply more fun, which means you'll ride them more, and that's worth a couple hundred bucks any day.

2) *Your level of investment should match your level of interest . . . long term. How you answered Question 2 will help provide your final price check. If you chose:*

A. No need to second-guess yourself. Leave the bike shop with a new ride and a smile.

B. Weigh your options a little. If you're not sure this cycling thing will stick, consider buying a good bike that you can improve upon if you end up really loving it. If you buy a frame made of high-quality material (aluminum, titanium, high-quality steel) you can always upgrade to lighter wheels and high-end shifting, braking, and other components.

C. They say you never forget how to ride a bike, and even if you drift away from the sport, you can always come back to it easily. Buy the bike you love, and enjoy it today.

M Y   N E W   B I K E !

Jot down the answers to your Bike Finder test for a snapshot of
the bike you should buy.

Part I:
My bike type:

_____

(e.g., road bike, mountain bike, or hybrid)

Part II:
My price range:

_____

(e.g., $2,000, enthusiast road bike)

Part III
My setup should be:

_____

(e.g., relaxed; I'm more comfortable in an upright position)

Part IV:
My components should be:

_____

(e.g., top-of-the-line; I want my bike to be the best it can be)

YOUR BEST BIKE SHOP EXPERIENCE

True story: Recently, I offered to help a very good friend of mine buy her first "real" bike. She'd been commuting around town on an old box-store bike and wanted a light, nimble road bike to take exploring around our large network of Pennsylvania farm roads. Joyce is tall, blond, soft-spoken, and in her mid-forties. She's also very smart, has a lot of money, and doesn't mind buying the best. She came that day prepared to part with a few grand to buy a top-of-the-line bike. But the sales guys at the first bike shop we went to will never know that, because they were jerks.

We walked in. They looked her up and down, heard the lack of experience in her voice, and vaguely pointed to a bike or two before leaving her to her own devices. She was feeling conciliatory (as women too often do), but I refused to let her drop a dime with them. We went a few miles down the road to another shop where they spent the better part of an hour offering advice and guiding her in the right direction. She left with a $2,500 Trek, $300 worth of accessories, and a big smile. The moral of this story: shop around. If a bike shop feels like a boys-only treehouse where you need to know the secret code words to get attention, leave. But don't march into the nearest Wal-Mart. A good bike shop is worth the hunt and shouldn't be too hard to find (there are a few bad apples in the bunch, but most are great). Unlike department stores, where the salespeople generally know squat about cycling and you'll get zero service, bike store employees are knowledgeable and will be happy to provide years of assistance as you grow with the sport.

Like a good marriage, a positive bike shop experience takes two. Your job is to help them help you—and their job is to do just that. Below are some tips for having your best bike shop experience.

EXPLORE ONLINE

I don't recommend buying a bike online. You need to see, feel, touch, and ride a bike before you buy it. Also, when you buy from a catalog or the Internet, the bike will arrive in a box, requiring at least some assembly, instead of being ready to ride. You'll likely have more of a hassle returning it to the cyberstore than you would to your local bike shop, should something go wrong.

I *do* recommend doing lots of research online. Once you have a general idea of what type of bike you want, the Internet is a great place to start exploring your options. By researching road racing bikes or commuting bikes online, you can learn what brands are out there and what specific bikes you might want to buy. Many bike company Web sites will also have "dealer finder" tools to help you locate a shop in your area that carries their brands.

CALL AROUND

Bike shops are like car dealerships. Each carries specific makes and models (e.g., your local Bike Line may carry Trek and Cannondale while Action Wheels down the road deals only in Jamis and Kona). Call ahead to see what the shop carries. Also ask if they specialize in a specific bike style. A shop that specializes in road bikes won't have a good selection of off-road machines and vice versa.

BRING YOUR NOTES

After you've done your homework, write everything down and bring it to the bike shop, so your mind doesn't turn to mush the moment you walk in the door.

GET SIZED UP

Like blue jeans and dresses, all bike brands fit a little differently, even in the same size. Have the shop measure your inseam and torso length to determine which sizes in the specific brands you're interested in are right for you. Once you've found a bike in the right size, the shop should also provide a basic bike fit to make sure your feet, hands, and butt are in their proper places. If they don't immediately offer one, ask them to help you make fit adjustments (moving the saddle and so forth).

TAKE YOUR TIME

Don't expect to buy a bike on your lunch hour. Give yourself a couple of hours to survey the inventory, choose a few models that look right, and take them on the road. (If the bike shop says no to test rides, go elsewhere; you can't be expected to buy a bike you haven't ridden.) Again, don't just noodle around the parking lot. Take the bike around the block. Sometimes a bike shop employee may be willing to accompany you, so you can ask questions as you ride.

The more you're investing in your bike, the longer you should expect the buying process to take. Buying a top-of-the-line road bike may require weeks of research and test rides. Purchasing a custom frame can take months. But it's worth the wait for a bike that may just last a lifetime.

COME DRESSED TO RIDE

Sounds obvious, but you'd be amazed how many women show up to buy a bike in snug jeans and sandals. You can't possibly know if a bike is comfortable if you can't bend forward to reach the bars without your rear end peeping out or your shoes flopping off. You don't have to come kitted up for the Tour de France, but wear clothes, such as yoga pants if you don't yet own bike shorts, you can move in.

ASK ABOUT PARTS SWAPS

Not all bodies are proportioned to bike manufacturers' specifications. A bike shop should be willing to swap minor parts (like a handlebar stem, which affects how far you need to reach to grasp the bars) to ensure proper fit.

KNOW THEIR SERVICE POLICY

Ask what kind of service plan the shop offers. A year of free tune-ups is a good starting point. Bikes typically need a lot of small adjustments during the first few months of riding as the cables stretch and components break in.

AVOID HAGGLING

Buying a bike isn't like buying a car, where you're expected to try to pay something other than sticker price. The profit margin on a bike is small, so shops can't afford to offer big discounts. Many shops will toss in a couple of niceties (e.g., a water bottle and some small accessories) for shopping with them. You also might be offered a percentage discount if you get completely outfitted with new bike and clothes. But the bottom line is you should expect to pay the listed price. You'll get your money's worth in good service down the road.

LAST STOP: THE CYBERSTORE

Again, I'm not in favor of online bike shopping. But I recognize that sometimes there's little alternative, especially for people buying in the high-end bike categories where you may be interested in a make and model that only a few shops in the country carry. (However, note that many high-end bikes refuse to sell online and are available through licensed dealers only.) If you must go into cyberspace, here's what you should know:

BEWARE eBay

Experts estimate that about 65% of bikes and bike parts sold on this online auction site are literally hot off the press—stolen. I've been at races and bike events where brand-new bikes are stolen en masse. I know guys who have gotten great deals on eBay only to have a brand-new, obviously stolen bike arrive. I'm not blaming eBay. They can't police billions of transactions and know where every item of merchandise originated. But I would be *very* cautious buying a bike from there.

BUY DIRECT

Some companies, like Seven Cycles, sell directly to consumers. In those cases, you're sure to know exactly what you're getting.

TALK TO SOMEONE

When ordering online, try to speak to an actual human being. Be sure you clearly understand their delivery and exchange policies. In many cases, you will be responsible for shipping charges if you are returning a bike for reasons other than defects.

CONSIDER JUST FRAME AND FORK

If you're upgrading, consider buying just the frame and fork online. That way you can take the bare-bones bike skeleton to your local bike shop and build up a bike with components that work best for the kind of riding you will be doing. This takes a little longer, but you'll get the best of both worlds by buying the bike brand you want while still making sure you get the right fit and building a relationship with your local bike shop.

PROPER BIKE FIT

Entire books have been written on this single topic, because good bike fit is essential for maximum cycling joy. The bottom line is you shouldn't be uncomfortable. Nothing should feel stretched out, scrunched up, or unnatural. Your bike shop will help set you up initially, but as you ride longer distances, you may find little aches or pains cropping up here or there. Those are almost always signs that something doesn't fit quite right. Don't be afraid to make minor adjustments. You'll be surprised what a difference even a centimeter shift here or there can make.

The following are some fundamentals to get you started. These adjustments should be enough for recreational, moderate-mileage riding. If you plan on racing or doing long touring, I would recommend a professional bike fitting.

SEAT HEIGHT

This determines your reach from the seat to the pedals. In the fully extended position, your leg should have a slight bend in the knee (rather than being completely locked out). Your pelvis should stay stable on the saddle, not rock from side to side as you pedal. Seat height is important not just for producing power as you pedal but for knee comfort. If the seat is too low, you put undue pressure on your knees, causing pain in the front of the knee. If the seat is too high, you end up overextending and getting nagging aches in the back of the knee.

FOOT PLACEMENT

Whether you ride in special cycling shoes or your sneakers, you want the ball of your foot to be placed directly over the pedal spindle (the extension where the pedal connects to the crank arms) for maximum power transfer.

SADDLE POSITION

Your saddle not only moves up and down but also forward and back (you'll hear this referred to as *fore* and *aft*). To check for proper fore and aft positioning, place your feet on the pedals and position them so they are parallel to the ground in the three-o'clock and nine-o'clock positions. The front of your forward knee should be directly over the ball of the forward foot. (Someone can drop a line from your knee to your foot to check.) You also want to make sure your saddle is level, not pointing up or dipping down.

HANDLEBAR REACH

You can position your handlebar closer or farther away from you by changing the stem (the piece that connects the handlebar to the top of the bike) to one that is longer or shorter. You also can adjust your reach by adding spacers between the stem and the head tube (the tube where the fork comes through from the bottom). This will raise the handlebars, so you don't have to bend as far. Where you place your handlebars depends on how flexible you are. Don't feel like you must hunker down as low as you can go despite discomfort because the bike comes set up in a super "aero" low handlebar position. You should be able to reach all the hand positions on your bars, including the lowest "down in the drops," without feeling stretched out. If you can't, work with the shop to adjust it to your comfort.

BUTT, SERIOUSLY, YOU *CAN* BE COMFORTABLE ON A BIKE SEAT

All the proper fitting in the world isn't going to help if you're sitting on the wrong saddle. No bike part is as personal or as important as the seat—known as the "saddle." It's the part that cradles your most sensitive tissues, and there's no getting around it. If it's not right, it's a pain in the butt (and then some!).

The first rule of saddle fit is that it's supposed to support your sit bones, not your whole butt. Many a first-time bike buyer is aghast with horror when she lays eyes (but not butt cheeks) on the skinny saddles most bikes sport. Even if you have more booty than the pirates of the Caribbean, you can be perfectly comfy on a slim saddle, so long as it supports your sit bones—the ends of the pelvic bones that protrude when we sit down. Because women have wider hips than men, these bones tend to be farther apart. Women-specific saddles flare more in the back to accommodate this anatomical difference.

While the rear of the saddle supports your sit bones, the nose (front) allows you to control the bike with your legs and supports *some* of your body weight. That *some* part is very important. Your girl parts should not be smooshed, go numb, or be subject to chafing. First, be sure your position and fit are right. Reaching too far to the handlebars is one of the primary culprits behind sore crotches. Next, check that your sit bones are properly planted at the rear of the saddle. If both fit and positioning check out and you're still feeling too much pressure on your girl parts, look for a saddle with a more forgiving nose. Some models actually have cutaways in the nose to relieve pressure, while others incorporate a dugout channel that runs the length of the seat. Try a few designs to find the one that works for you. Word to the wise: Some riders assume that a cushy saddle will solve all their problems so they make a beeline to the gel saddles. Heavy padding may feel comfortable at first, but as you ride, your sit bones will sink into the padding, increasing the pressure on your crotch. Stick with more moderate cushioning.

Finally, even the most satisfying seat may leave your tush a little tender after your first few rides. This will disappear after a couple of weeks in the saddle. As you ride more, your butt muscles become denser (firm butt: good thing!) and will support you pain free even for long rides. To minimize this problem, start with thirty- or forty-five-minute rides and gradually lengthen the amount of time you spend in the saddle to give your butt time to "break in" to the sport.

WOMEN-SPECIFIC DESIGNS

Once the domain of a few niche manufacturers, women-specific bikes are now a staple for all the major players in the cycling market. Why? Because bike companies finally realize that women are not just small men with boobs. I'm not even remotely petite, but the women-specific bikes I have ridden from Specialized, Trek, Terry, Santa Cruz, Giant and Cannondale have been instantly more comfortable than their unisex brethren. The difference is multifactorial, but it boils down to:

LESS REACH

Women's arms and hands are proportionately shorter than men's, and women often have longer legs and relatively shorter torsos. That means, even if you're the same height as a man, you may be stretched out too far over the same bike that fits him like a glove. The result: pain and discomfort, most notably in the low back, shoulders, neck, and/or hands. You also can't produce as much power in this compromised position. Women's bikes tend to have shorter top tubes that reduce the reach. The kicker is that if you're new to the sport, you may not notice feeling stretched out (I know I never did) on a unisex bike (and maybe you're not). That's why test-riding different bikes is essential. Good fit is hard to describe in black and white, but you know it when you feel it.

LIGHTER IN THE REAR

Women's pelvic structure is wider (relative to our shoulders) and shallower than men's. Our sit bones are farther apart and angle out more than men's. Our pelvises also tilt back, so our lovely butts curve out farther. We also store more "fuel" back there. This apple-cheek effect carves a sexy profile in blue jeans but can make us bottom heavy on a bike, which compromises the bike's ability to stop and steer, not to mention makes for a tender tush (and labia) after a long day in the saddle. Women-specific bikes combine taller head tubes (the tube that holds the handlebar) with shorter top tubes to bring the handlebars and saddle closer together for more balanced weight distribution, giving you more control steering through corners, putting more power into your pedals, and generally allowing you to maneuver the bike better. Women's bikes also come equipped with flared, female-specific saddles, so your sit bones sit right where they're supposed to.

BETTER GRIP

The WNBA uses a smaller ball for good reason—our hands aren't as big as men's. Women-specific bikes recognize this fact with narrower handlebars, which put your hands in the right place, reducing shoulder and neck ache, and shorter-reach brakes and shifter levers so you can work these essential levers without undue hand fatigue.

EASY RIDING

Depending on the manufacturer, women-specific bikes may also have shorter cranks (the levers that attach the pedals to the bike), lower gearing (for easier pedaling), and even smaller wheels, all of which are geared to give smaller women a better ride. Obviously there's a lot to be said for women-specific designs, so by all means test-ride a few and feel the difference for yourself. It may give you a whole new perspective on bicycling comfort. Or you may shrug and buy a unisex bike that fits you better. It's just nice to finally have the choice.

GO WITH YOUR GUT

A few years ago a friend of the family fired me an e-mail with a picture of a bike he was thinking about buying. "What do you think?" he asked innocently. In retrospect, I should have said, "Great! Buy it!" because it was a perfectly fine bike for the kind of riding he'd be doing. Instead, I got all excited and sent him half a dozen links to other bikes I thought were better as well as a dog-eared copy of *Bicycling* magazine's Buyer's Guide replete with Post-it notes and circled choices.

He never bought a bike. The moral of this story is that, as you've learned, there are a *lot* of bikes to choose from. The choices can be overwhelming, and it's easy to find yourself in a state of analysis paralysis. That's when it's time to just go with your gut. When you just can't make up your mind, buy the bike you're most attracted to without giving it too much more thought. It's better to have an "imperfect" bike to ride than a perfect one that exists only in your mind.

3

Gearing Up

*All the Right Stuff
for Riding Better
and Looking Great*

Fair warning: You're going to go into your bike shop for a bike and you're going to leave with a bag of stuff and a Visa bill both bigger than you expected. Make peace with it now. Better yet, have fun with it. This is an investment in yourself, in your physical and mental health. Every time you go for a ride, it's like a mini-vacation. So it's definitely worth a few extra bucks up front to have a really good time over and over again.

As you've no doubt figured out, bicycling is a gear-oriented sport. You need gear (a bike, helmet, water bottle) to get started. And there's an endless slew of gear being shot out by manufacturers every year that promises to help you to ride longer and stronger and to have more fun. What do you need? What might you want? What can you definitely live without (at least for a while)? That's what this chapter is all about. For simplicity's sake, we'll break it down into two categories: gear for your bike and gear for your body.

GEAR UP YOUR BIKE

As an invincible teen, I thought nothing of riding ten miles out into the country without a spare tube (or ID . . . or water . . . or a helmet . . . what were my parents thinking?). Never once did I have a flat tire. Never even thought about it. After college, I walked into a bike shop, bought a cheap bike, and took it on a long ride outside of Philadelphia. Seven miles out, I flatted. I was dumbfounded . . . and clueless. I found a pay phone (no cell phones then) and called the shop. *I have a flat tire.* "Uh, okay. Do you have a tube?" *No.* "Do you have a patch?" *No.* "Do you have any tools?" *No.* And being new to the area I didn't have any friends or family to call, either. Guess who walked home, grumbling and swearing the whole way? The moral of this story: Don't do what I did; you'll feel stupid about it for years. Here's what you need . . . and a few things you may want.

BOTTLE CAGE/WATER BOTTLE

Most bikes come equipped with two water bottle mounts, places on the frame where you can easily attach a cage that will hold bottles. The cages themselves, however, come separately, as do the water bottles that go in them. Pick up two of each so you can carry all the fluids you need for a long ride.

SADDLEBAG

This is a small bag that straps onto the rails beneath your seat for carrying spare tubes (see below), cash, and what have you. It's a great up-front investment, because you can pack it with your emergency items, nestle it under your saddle, and forget about it until you need it.

FIX-IT KIT

Flats happen. But they're no big deal if you have the tools (and know-how—more on that in Chapter 10, "Get Your Hands Dirty") to fix them. You'll need:

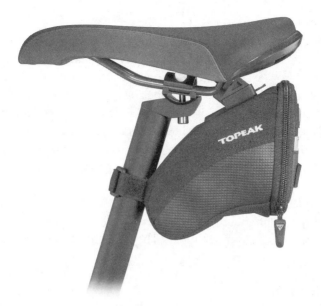

Most saddlebags are designed to tuck under the seat.
Photo courtesy of Topeak

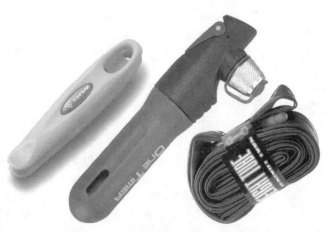

A saddlebag typically carries a spare tube, tire levers, and a CO_2 cartridge
to refill the new tire.
Photo courtesy of Topeak, Mitch Mandel/RODALE

Inner tube

Inside your tires are inflatable tubes. Get yourself a few spares and carry one with you at all times. They come in different sizes for different size wheels, so check the outside of your tires for the correct dimensions (the bike shop should be able to tell at a glance what you need). Tubes also come with one of two different types of inflation valve, Presta or Schrader. Presta are slimmer, easier to inflate, and are the standard on most road bikes. Go with those. Schrader valves are thicker and heavier, so many cyclists avoid them.

Tire levers

Bike tires fit snugly on their rims. You'll need tire levers to pry them off to change inner tubes. They're light, cheap, and usually come in sets of three.

Patch kit

These small kits can be a lifesaver if you get unlucky and have two flats in one day. You can choose between glueless patches, which you use by simply peeling off the backing and sticking them to the tire like a Band-Aid, or patches that come with a small tube of glue that you use to stick on the patch. Obviously, glueless patches are quicker and easier to apply, but they really don't last as long or work as well as regular patches, which adhere forever and leave your tire as good as new.

Pump or CO2 cartridge

You'll need an air source to pump up your tire when the flat is fixed. You have several options: a frame pump, a mini-pump, CO2 cartridges, or a combination CO2/pump system. A frame pump attaches to the underside of your top tube and inflates your tire with a few easy strokes. Problem is they don't fit on all frames, so be sure to check before you buy. A mini-pump will easily fit in a pocket or saddlebag, but be warned it takes a million little strokes to inflate your tire (also note you usually need to top off the tire with a floor pump when you get home). CO2 cartridges are small metal containers of compressed air that you attach to a special device that unleashes the air into your tire. They're amazingly quick. But if you have more flats than cartridges, you're stuck. That's why I like a CO_2 mini-pump. It's a mini-pump with CO_2 option, so your bases are fully covered. It's also small enough to stuff into a saddlebag.

Multi-tool

Truth be told, you can probably put this item in your "to buy later" pile, because if you have a mechanical problem big enough to warrant one, chances are good you'll just use another, easier-to-use tool: your cell phone. That said, I carry one as do most of the riders I know. Multi-tools are the Swiss Army knives of cycling—they're screwdrivers, Allen wrenches, bottle openers, chain tools, and more all wrapped up in a portable package. I've used mine about five times in all the years I've been riding, but I was very happy I had it each of those times. If you do put off buying a multi-tool, consider buying a few Allen wrenches instead. These come in handy for tightening bolts, including those that hold your bottle cages on, that can occasionally come loose on a ride.

Duct tape

Tear off a few inches of duct tape, roll it around a golf tee or small pencil, and carry it with you. I once used a strip to fasten down a dangling water bottle cage when one of the bolts came loose (and then went missing). In a pinch, you *might* be able to fix a small puncture in your tire with it (at least to get you home). You never know when it might come in handy.

LUBE

Bicycle chains need regular lubing to keep them running smoothly and protect your gears from premature wear. There's a mind-boggling array of lubes to choose from (see the "Choices, Choices" box, page 291). Your bike shop can steer you in the right direction. One nice feature to look for is self-cleaning, which means the lube acts like a solvent that cleans the chain of debris and old lube while it lubricates.

FLOOR PUMP

Believe it or not, your tires will lose air even if you never run over glass or otherwise flatten them. It just ever so slowly seeps out. Don't try using your mini-pump to inflate your tires on a regular basis. Get a standard floor pump (one that stands upright on the floor) to keep in the garage and pump your tires before every other ride or so. Floor pumps are quick and easy to use and have gauges that tell you your tire pressure; many also have convenient markings right on the gauge indicating appropriate pressure for road, mountain, and hybrid bikes.

LOCK

A bike lock is optional depending on where you're riding and how you'll be using your bike. Recreational riders who leave their bikes unattended (usually with the rest of their friends' bikes) only for short stretches to grab coffee or water refills generally don't fuss over bike locks. Urban commuters carry one wherever they go. Look for a sturdy lock with enough cable to secure your bike frame to a bike rack, signpost, small tree, or other street fixture. If you ride in a city where bikes are a favored target of thieves, carry two locks: a chain to secure the frame and back wheel to a rack and a U-lock (a lock shaped like a U with a removable bar across the top) to lock the front wheel to the frame. Many city commuters also attach a small permanent chain to attach the saddle to the bike. (It's no fun riding if your saddle goes missing!)

COMPUTER

Optional, but very fun and rather addictive, the cycling computer is a sophisticated odometer for your bike. A small screen that affixes to your handlebar, the computer speaks to a little sensor you attach to your front wheel. Together they tell you all sorts of interesting facts including how fast you're pedaling, how far you went, what your average and maximum speeds were, how long you rode, and so on. Fancy models even gauge your altitude and read the outside temperature. If you plan on doing bike tours and large charity rides, you should go ahead and spring for a computer right away, because you often need to know your mileage to follow the cue sheets provided for those types of events. If you're just going to be joyriding, a computer can wait, if you choose to buy one at all.

If you're riding for weight loss or weight maintenance, consider purchasing a computer that works with a heart rate monitor (see "Listen to Your Heart," page 96), which along with all the other stats on your ride includes calories burned. Keeping track of the energy you use and matching it to the calories you consume is the ticket to quick and healthy weight loss.

CLIPLESS PEDALS

If your bike didn't come with clipless pedals (see page 24), consider investing in a pair. It's not a priority-one item, but on rides longer than, say, five or ten miles, they enhance your enjoyment tenfold. Why? Because they hold your feet securely to the pedals, so all the power generated from your spinning legs goes directly into moving you forward. You save energy while going farther and faster. You can use toe clips and straps, which strap the top of your foot to your pedal, but they're pretty uncomfortable and ultimately harder to get in and out of. Once you go clipless, you'll never go back. (We'll talk more about how to ride clipless pedals later.)

Now, I take that all back if most of your riding is commuting where there's a lot of stopping and starting and quick footwork involved. In those situations, being firmly attached to your pedals is a distinct disadvantage and potentially dangerous. Better to just ride flat pedals with some very loose toe clips, so you can maximize your pedal stroke while having your feet mostly free.

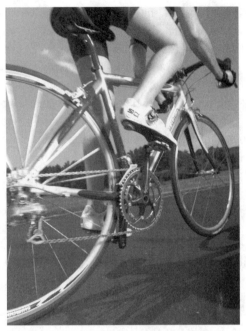

Shoes that "clip in," or attach to the pedal, give you more power on the down and up stroke.
Photo by Liz Reap

GEAR UP YOUR BODY

Long gone are the days when women were forced to buy small men's clothes that fit nowhere and flattered nothing. Thanks to an active women's clothing revolution started by such companies as Terry twenty years ago, women's cycling attire is downright cute. With all the flirty prints, body-shaping cuts, tanks, wraps, skorts, and jackets, you'll be tempted to wear some of it off the bike as well as on.

Some women may ask if they even need cycling-specific attire. Aside from padded shorts, which have an obvious functional advantage, why pay more for shirts, glasses, gloves, and the like? Because cycling places very different demands on your clothing than running, hiking, skiing, or other outdoor sports. For one, you're bent forward from the waist; this rules out wearing top layers as in other sports, which will ride up and expose your lower back the instant you reach forward for the bars. Cyclists also have very still upper bodies that bear the brunt of the elements, so it's important to have some wind protection in all the right places, which cycling clothes provide.

Yes, cycling-specific clothing tends to be pricey, but it lasts a long time. I have jerseys that have stood up to a decade of wear and tear. And there are always year-end sales. With that, here's a look at the clothing and accessories that will sweeten your riding experience:

HELMET

Gotta have one. Period. No matter how expert a rider you are, a squirrel can still run out from the roadside and send you tumbling to the pavement. Why tempt fate? Put a lid on your head and keep your brain safe from harm's way. Today's helmets are light, stylish, and extremely well ventilated. Some women's models even come ponytail compatible, meaning there's special space in the back to accommodate your fastened mane. Look for a helmet with a locking retention system that allows you to get a snug, comfortable fit. The helmet should fit level on your head, sitting right above your eyebrows in the front. Adjust the side straps so they form a V around your ears and tighten them so the straps connect snugly under your chin, allowing just enough room for two fingers to slip through. The helmet should stay put when you shake your head.

When you start shopping for helmets you'll notice that the price points vary dramatically. It's reasonable for a woman to wonder if that fancy $275 helmet protects her head and its valuable contents better than the bucket-style lid that costs just $35. The real deal is any helmet sold in the United States must meet the U.S. Consumer Product Safety Commission standard (you'll see a CPSC sticker somewhere on the inside), so any helmet will absorb impact and buffer your brains from a bad crash. Pricier helmets tend to be lighter, more stylish, and have better ventilation to keep your head cooler. But the Consumers Union (the relentless testers behind *Consumer Reports*) recently ranked two helmets by Bell (the Citi and Slant) as their Best Buys for providing very good protection for just $45 to $50.

GLASSES

Most any sunglasses will block dangerous UV rays and make it easier to see on brilliant sunny days, but cycling-specific shades are shatterproof, which is essential should a rock fly up and hit the lenses. Many sport-specific sunglasses also come with cool features like interchangeable lenses (light lenses for overcast days, dark ones for cloudless rides), rubberized nose grips to keep the glasses firm on your face, and wraparound lenses for 100% protection from rays, bugs, and debris.

If you're a mountain biker who rides on tree-shaded trails or a commuter who rides in dim light or darkness, you'll also need some glasses with clear lenses to provide protection without diminishing your already compromised vision. In that case, you might want to investigate some of the sport-specific glasses with interchangeable lenses, as many offer clear lenses as an option. (I have a colleague who simply wears safety glasses. They're light and shatterproof and cost about $8. They won't win you many style points, but they get the job done.)

SHORTS AND TIGHTS

Cycling shorts provide extra padding (called chamois) where you need it most, under your bum and tender nether regions. Women-specific shorts have chamois that are specially cut to fit the female anatomy. You can buy regular shorts with elastic-band waists, or "bibs," which have suspender-like shoulder straps and ride higher on your torso (be warned they make it hard to pee quickly, since you have to squirm out of your jersey and take down the straps to pull down the shorts). Cycling-specific shorts are made of wicking, quick-drying material to keep you dry and comfortable. For colder weather riding you can buy full-length tights or knickers (capri-length tights) that keep your knees from being cold. (Most riders keep their knees covered until at least 65 degrees; warm knees are less likely to fall prey to aches and pains.)

Wouldn't be caught dead wearing Lycra in public? Opt for a skort, a pair of bike shorts hidden under a skirt. "Serious cyclists" may snicker (they can be snobs), but they're surprisingly comfy to ride in (I've even raced in one) and will make even the most modest pedaler proud. Oh, and here's an insider's tip: You don't wear underwear under cycling shorts. They're designed to be worn bareback. Otherwise you risk chafing, sores, and visible panty lines.

JERSEY

Save the cotton tees for the gym. For cycling, you'll want a special shirt called a jersey, which comes equipped with a zipper in the front for cooling off when the going gets hot and pockets in the back for stashing a few fig bars, spare cash, and your cell phone. Cycling jerseys tend to be brightly colored so motorists can spot you easily, and they're made of wicking material to keep you dry. They're also tailored to be longer in the back, so your skin isn't exposed in the bent-over cycling position.

GLOVES

Padded cycling gloves are a good idea even in the summertime because they absorb bumps and vibration from the road for increased comfort and protect your palms in case you fall. They're not a must-have (you'll see plenty of riders spinning around without them) but definitely a should have. If you're just learning to ride on clipless pedals (when your chances of falling over in the parking lot are high), you should definitely have some hand protection.

You can buy both fingerless (for warm weather riding) and

full-fingered gloves. If you plan on doing a lot of winter riding, invest in lobster gloves (mitten-glove hybrids that bundle your first and second and third and fourth fingers together for added warmth). They're super toasty and can keep your fingers from freezing in even sub-twenty temps.

SHOES

If you have clipless pedals, you need cycling shoes, which accommodate cleats that attach to the pedals. Cycling shoes have stiff soles that ensure all the energy from your pedaling transfers into propelling the bike down the road. Stiff soles also prevent your feet from fatiguing from bending and flexing with every revolution, which can result in arch pain and other foot problems.

The type of shoes you choose depends on the type of riding you do. Mountain bike shoes come with what are known as recessed cleats. These shoes have a normal tread and the cleat is nestled below tread level, so they're easy to walk in—a plus when you have to hike your bike through unrideable sections of a trail. Most road bike shoes, especially high-performance road shoes, have perfectly flat soles (they're also lighter and stiffer), so the cleat protrudes from the ball of your foot, which makes walking in them pretty awkward. It's a good idea to match your shoes to your riding; however, if you're going to do both on- and off-road riding and can spring for only one pair of shoes, go for mountain shoes. It's easier to ride mountain bike shoes on the road than to hike around in road shoes.

SOCKS

Yep, they make special cycling socks, too. Truth be told, you don't need them (though they sure do come in some very cute colors and designs). But do be sure to wear a merino wool or synthetic (Coolmax, etc.) athletic-style sock that is designed to wick moisture away from your feet to keep them dry.

CHAMOIS CREAM

I'll never forget my first ride with an ex-pro woman and watching her scoop a golf ball–size glob of Noxzema out of a jar and shove it down her shorts. Uncomfortable as it looked, she knew what she was doing. On long rides, a slippery barrier between your skin and your chamois prevents chafing that causes tenderness, hot spots, and saddle sores. You can use Noxzema, A and D ointment, even Bag Balm (an ointment designed for cows' udders), or pick up one of the specialty chamois creams at the bike shop. It's not necessary for short rides, but if you are heading out for hours in the saddle, a little butter on your butt is just what the doctor ordered.

VEST

Underappreciated, but oh so handy, a cycling vest should be on your wish list (cycling clothes make great gifts in case you blanch at buying everything for yourself). Because your upper body is fairly inactive and you generate a lot of wind when you ride (since you're slicing through the air), it's easy for your torso to get cold even on a fairly warm spring day. They're also great protection against stiff breezes and chilly descents. Look for one that has wind and water protection on the front and mesh in the back to prevent overheating.

ARM/LEG WARMERS

Arm warmers rank near the iPod on the list of smartest inventions. Hyperbolic? Maybe. But you won't think so when you realize that you don't have to worry about whether you should wear long or short sleeves for a ride that starts at nine a.m. (when it might be 60 degrees) and ends at eleven (when it can easily be ten or fifteen degrees warmer), because you can have the best of both worlds with a pair of portable sleeves. Leg warmers are nice too, but most riders use them considerably less often since you actually have to get off the bike to peel them off (unless you're a *really* good bike handler!), while arm warmers can be peeled off and stuffed in a pocket while you're rolling down the road. Do you need them? No. Will you love them? Yes.

JACKET

Cycling-specific jackets are designed to keep you comfortable in cool, windy, and/or rainy conditions. They're also designed with extra material in the back to keep your low back and butt dry when you're bent over the handlebars. How much outer protection you need depends on your climate and whether or not you plan on riding if it's cold and/or wet enough to need a jacket. If you live in one of those states where the weather changes from sunny to stormy every ten minutes or so, a lightweight waterproof windbreaker is a must. Ditto if you plan on doing multi-day charity rides where riding in chilly or rainy weather isn't optional. Otherwise, you can probably put a cycling jacket on your "buy later" wish list.

The same philosophy applies to winter jackets or heavy winter jerseys. If you plan on riding when the temperatures head south, cold weather attire is a must. I have a winter jersey that's so warm I can wear it over a tank top in thirty-degree weather and be perfectly comfortable for the whole ride. Look for microfiber (fine fleece) to keep you warm, windblock to protect you from arctic breezes, and other nice features such as fitted cuffs to keep the wind from traveling up your arms and zipper vents to cool off if you get too toasty.

BASE LAYER

Some riders never dream of going out without a base layer—a thin undershirt you wear under your jersey to wick away moisture and provide an extra layer of skin protection should you have an accident. But they're completely optional and women usually have a jog bra on anyway. The only time you really need one is when the temperatures dip. During chilly winter months, I swear by a long-sleeve silk turtleneck to keep my core cozy and warm.

HYDRATION PACK

Sometimes called CamelBaks, after the most popular brand of hydration pack, these are small backpacks that typically hold fifty to one hundred ounces of water as well as assorted odds and ends, such as car keys, food, tools, cell phone, and anything else you might cart along for a day of riding. A CamelBak is an excellent way to carry water on mountain bike rides when you're often out in remote places where it's not so easy to refill water bottles. Most road riders don't use hydration packs, with the exception of long-distance cyclists (who need to carry lots and lots of stuff) and for multi-day tours (again, where you need to carry lots of stuff and you may end up riding long stretches with nowhere to stop and refill bottles).

LAYER LIKE A WEDDING CAKE

To stay warm during cool-weather rides you're better off wearing multiple layers than trying to wear a single thick layer. Layers trap your body heat between them, so you stay warmer. You can also remove a layer should the temperature rise unexpectedly. Your layers should be made of wicking materials (such as polypropylene) that pull moisture away from your skin to keep you dry.

Layering for a thirty-five-degree ride would look something like:

Base layer: A long- or short-sleeve undershirt
Middle layer: A long- or short-sleeve cycling jersey, depending on the weight of your top layer.
Top layer: A shell or jacket that's made from material that provides wind protection.

BOOTIES

Cycling shoes are well ventilated to keep your feet cool. Great for the summer, not so much during colder months. For cold weather riding, invest in a pair of booties—covers that slip over your cycling shoes and provide an added layer of insulation. You also can buy lightweight rain booties to keep your feet dry in soggy riding conditions.

FIND YOUR STYLE

How much cycling-specific gear you need is ultimately a personal preference. Two of my best friends are polar opposites in this category. Christine often shows up without socks or gloves, sometimes even sporting a Swiss-cheesy threadbare T-shirt that's flapping in the breeze. Beth always arrives decked out in a stylish, color-coordinated Lycra ensemble. Both are killer riders. Both love the sport. Both are a ton of fun to ride with. They just approach it differently. Take your time getting to know the sport. The longer you ride and the more miles you put in, the clearer your understanding of what you personally need, and what you don't, will be.

4

How to Ride

There's More to It Than Just Spinning Your Wheels

A few years back I volunteered to help lead a local charity ride called the Spirit of Women. As I watched hundreds of women spin down our rural Pennsylvania roads on their dusted-off Schwinns, I quickly realized that though nearly every one of them knew how to pedal a bike, many had no idea how to actually ride one.

Case in point: I pedaled up next to a woman who was bobbing and weaving so much as she struggled to crest a small rise in the road I feared she might topple over (or take out another rider). I looked down at her bike and noticed she was in her hardest gear. She looked pretty unhappy, so I offered a little advice: "Why don't you shift down? You're in your hardest gear."

Puzzled silence.

"Your gears," I repeated. "You're in your hardest. That's why you're having such a hard time on this hill."

More puzzled silence, punctuated by a deeply furrowed brow.

I pointed at her shifter and told her to push it.

Click. Click. Her legs spun faster. An amazed smile crossed her face. "I always wondered what those did!"

The whole ride she'd been suffering, counting down the miles 'til she could get off her bike, thinking what terrible shape she was in. And all it took was a change of gears to shift her perspective and convert her to a cyclist.

It's not a knock on her. No one ever showed her how her bike worked, and she didn't want to "screw it up" by flipping levers willy-nilly. That may be an extreme example, but it's more common than you think.

LEARN THE ESSENTIALS

Even women who have a basic understanding of how their bikes work don't always know how to really work their bikes when riding up steep hills, sweeping through corners, or coming to quick stops. Heck, even seasoned pros can benefit from brushing up on some of those skills. That's where this chapter comes in. You'll learn how to shift smartly, brake evenly, and maneuver your bike with skill, grace, and most important, confidence.

SHIFTING: DO IT EARLY AND OFTEN

Even people who know they have gears are often leery of using them. I was outside raking leaves the other day when my neighbor called me over. Scott is a sharp, athletic guy who could probably disassemble and reassemble my lawn mower in the time it takes me to start the darn thing. "Selene," he said. "What gear do you ride in?"

"Uh. All of them." I thought, *What do you mean?*

"I want you to put my bike in the right gear for me, and I'll just keep it there."

I explained that riding is easier and more fun when you use all your gears, because each one is designed to handle different grades and conditions.

I'm convinced that understanding shifting can mean the difference between loving and leaving the sport. Your bike has anywhere from eighteen to thirty gears, and you should use them liberally for maximum enjoyment. Your gears are designed to help you pedal with relative ease whether the road goes up, down, or remains perfectly flat. Here's how they work.

Gears are the same thing as "speeds." If you have two chainrings (the circular gears) in the front and ten cogs or gears in the back, you have a twenty-speed bike. When you shift, you move the chain from one chainring and/or gear to another. This makes pedaling easier or harder by shortening or lengthening the distance the bike moves forward with each rotation of the pedals. A big gear moves it farther per rotation, making it more difficult to pedal. A small gear moves it a shorter distance, making the effort easier.

Your lower gears are the easier gears; your higher gears are the harder ones. This *does not* mean that lower gears are for beginners and higher gears are for expert riders. All riders of all levels use easier and harder gears depending on the conditions, because the goal is to be able to pedal comfortably at all times. Some hybrids and mountain bikes have little windows on the shifters that tell you what number gear you're in, but you don't really need to know that. What matters is that you understand the concept of upshifting and downshifting. Quite simply: If you're pedaling uphill or into a strong wind and it feels difficult, shift down to an easier gear. If you're pedaling on a flat road, with the wind at your back, or downhill, and it feels too easy, shift up to a harder gear to cover more distance with every pedal stroke. As the road undulates, shift your gears to keep your effort consistent.

The shifter on the left side of your handlebars moves the chain from one chainring to the next. When you shift chainrings, the pedaling effort changes dramatically. If you have two chainrings, use the large one on flat roads (provided there's no strong headwind) or downhill and the small chainring on inclines and into the wind. If you have three chainrings, you'll likely spend most of your time in the middle ring, saving the big ring for very fast conditions

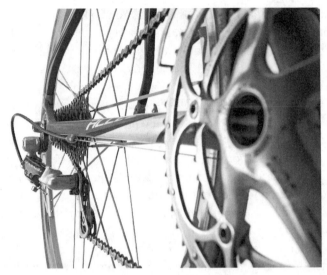

Shifting from small to big chainrings makes pedaling harder. Shifting from small to big cogs makes it easier. The big chainring/small rear cog combination (when the chain is to the far right in the front and back) is your highest (hardest) gear combination. The small chainring/biggest cog combination (when the chain is to the far left in the front and back) is your lowest (easiest) gear combination.

Most bikes have 2 to 3 big gear plates in front and 3 to 10 in back, which can offer you as many as 30 different gears to work with depending on the hills and valleys you encounter.

Photo by Mitch Mandel/RODALE

like downhill and your small ring for steep climbs or strong headwinds.

The shifter on the right side of your handlebars moves the chain from cog to cog in the back, which results in more subtle changes in pedaling effort. Think of this as fine-tuning. On undulating rides, you might park the chain on one ring but dance up and down the cogs throughout the entire ride. As you work through your gears, try to avoid "cross chaining," putting your chain at extreme angles. For example, putting the chain on the large (outside) chainring in the front and the large (inside) cog in the back. This stretches the chain and wears down the gears.

As you practice consciously shifting, your shifting will become more unconscious, until it's an automatic reflex that you barely register. One of the little joys I feel when riding with my longtime cycling friends is that we're all so attuned to our favorite routes that we practically shift in unison. It's like a chorus of clicks as we go up, up, up the usual climbs and another chorus down the other side.

How many "teeth" (the sharp pointy projections that the chain sits on) that each individual gear has also makes pedaling harder or easier. Your bike shop can make sure you have the right size gears for the kind of terrain you'll be riding; they can also help you switch your gears for specific events, like a Florida century or a Vermont tour.

That's the science of shifting. Shifting is also an art. It's about anticipating the change in conditions and shifting early, so your pedaling feels seamless instead of clunking through your gears as you shift on the toughest parts of climbs. With time and practice it will come.

SPINNING: FAST FEET STAVE OFF FATIGUE

Riding a bike is great exercise, but that doesn't mean it should feel like exercise every second of every ride. Most new riders (and plenty of "old" ones) make the mistake of being too macho. They feel like unless they're pushing hard on the pedals, they're really not doing anything. So they throw their bike into a high gear and mash away, fatiguing their muscles much more quickly than if they pedaled faster with less effort. This fast-pedaling technique is called spinning (the riding style the indoor cycling workout is named for), and it's the key to comfortable long-distance cycling.

Whenever your feet turn the pedals over one time through, it's called a revolution. Your cadence is how many revolutions you turn per minute while you ride. Determining your cadence is easy. Just count the number of times your right knee comes up for thirty seconds and multiply it by two. Many novice and occasional riders push larger gears at a lower cadence—somewhere around 50 to 70 RPM (revolutions per minute). Your ultimate goal is to increase your RPMs to 80 to 100. The magic number for most cyclists is right around 90.

Why so high? A few reasons. Most important, your muscles don't have to work as hard when you pedal in higher gears, so your legs stay fresher longer. It's also easier on your knees. Mashing a monster-size gear puts constant force on your knees and increases your risk of injury. Finally, it's easier to ride nimbly and respond quickly to changes in terrain and the speed of other riders when you're in a higher gear, because it takes less force to accelerate your bike.

All that said, learning to spin takes time. Though it's easier on your legs to ride in a high gear, it's harder from a fitness standpoint, at least initially. Spinning your legs at a quick cadence draws a lot of energy from your cardiovascular system. This is great, because you get really, really fit riding this way. But in the beginning it's a challenge because you'll find yourself getting winded and reaching for those bigger gears. The best way to learn to spin faster is to start slowly. Practice spinning faster than feels natural (but not higher than 100 RPM; you'll hit a diminishing point of returns) for ten or fifteen minutes on and off during the ride. As you get fitter, the fast pace will become more automatic.

It's also easier to spin when you have a smooth, pretty pedal stroke. That means your feet should be turning in perfect circles (as opposed to jamming down and bouncing up like a jackhammer) with equal amounts of pressure on the pedals throughout the entire revolution. You should picture yourself pulling your feet through the bottom of the pedal stroke (when your leg is extended) and up around the top. Your feet and ankles should stay strong and stable to help transfer the power. The action is similar to wiping mud off the soles of your shoes at the bottom of every pedal stroke. It also may help to concentrate on driving your knees toward the handlebars (as opposed to your feet pounding on the pedals). This helps lighten the pressure on the pedal coming up the back of the pedal stroke, so the one pushing down has less work to do. The end result is a more efficient pedal stroke with each leg doing less fatiguing work.

PEDALING: RIDING CLIPLESS

As discussed earlier, clipless pedals (meaning no toe clips or traps; you are actually "clipped" onto your pedals) are the way to go for optimum pedaling comfort and efficiency. Learning to ride that way takes some time, however, as you need to decide which pedal system is right for you and then learn to use it.

First is the choice of which clipless pedal system to buy. Most pedal manufacturers make clipless pedals for both road and mountain bikes. Though there are exceptions to this rule, mountain bike pedals tend to have a smaller cleat (the part that attaches to your shoe) but a larger pedal platform, and are designed to be easy to use even in dirty or muddy conditions. Road pedals often have larger cleats to provide a greater surface area to distribute the pedal pressure and keep your feet comfortable on long rides. The other distinguishing factor among pedals is the amount of "float," or lateral movement, they allow. Certain pedal systems lock your foot more tightly in place than others that allow more play. People with a history of knee problems generally require more float from their pedals. Your bike shop salesperson can help you find the pedal system that is best for your riding needs.

Once you have your pedals, you need to learn the art of clipping in and out. All pedal systems work essentially the same way. You step onto the pedal, applying pressure toe to heel to clip in, and you turn your heel out while pulling up to clip out. This takes practice—and I won't lie, you're bound to topple over once or twice because you don't clip out in time when coming to a stop. Practicing before you start riding can help you avoid this embarrassing scenario.

After attaching your pedals and cleats, place your bike next to a wall (either inside or outside) that you can easily prop yourself against while sitting on the saddle. Sit on the bike and lean against the wall with your right arm, leaving the right foot unclipped and resting on the pedal platform. With the left pedal in the down (six o'clock) position, practice clipping and unclipping with your left foot. Repeat until it comes easily. Flip the bike around and practice on the other side.

When you're ready, find a flat, wide-open space such as a grassy field or a quiet alley to practice on the fly. Ride fifty yards; then slowly come to a stop while clipping out. Keep practicing. As you become more comfortable, try stopping and clipping out more quickly. The more you practice, the more naturally it will come on the open road.

CORNERING: TAKE TURNS WITH CONFIDENCE

Your handlebars help steer your bike, but truly good cornering—that is, sweeping your bike through a sharp turn—is done with your body (and, man, is it a thing of beauty to behold!). Except at slow speeds (e.g., around 10 MPH), bikes, like motorcycles, turn by leaning. This is hands down one of the scariest skills for new riders, and even some longtime riders, to master. But with a little understanding and practice, you'll be able to take sharp turns with confidence. Here's what you need to know:

Get your hands in the drops

You want to keep your center of gravity low and your hands in close contact with the brakes when heading toward a turn. The best place for both is in the "drops," the lowest position on the handlebars.

Easy on the brakes

Some experts say you should never brake in a turn. That's like saying you should never squeeze a pimple. Pretty unrealistic. But just as you shouldn't pinch your face with abandon, you shouldn't come sailing in at high speed, panic, and grab two fistfuls of brake lever. The harder you brake, the more your bike wants to straighten out, which, as you can imagine, makes it tough to hold on to your line through a curve. It's also a surefire way to skid out and hit the pavement. Instead, try to feather the brakes lightly and scrub most of your speed before you enter the turn. Then turn with minimal, if any, braking.

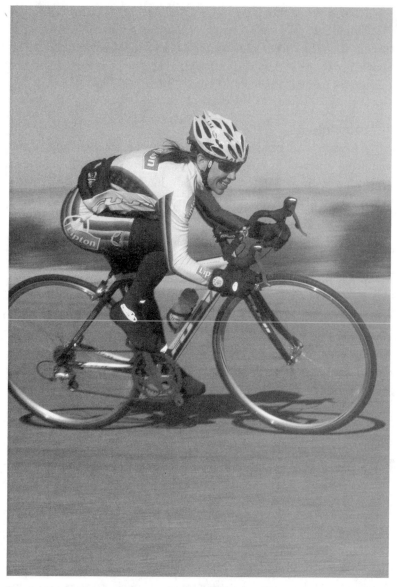

Flawless cornering includes angled pedals and a low, centered position on the bike.
Photo by Casey B. Gibson

Take a wide line

Think outside, inside, outside as you come into the corner. That is, come into the corner wide (but don't cross the yellow line!), cut the apex close to the inside, and exit wide. The goal is to ride as straight of a line as possible through the turn.

Lean into it

For wide, sweeping corners where you can see your line all the way from entry to exit, the easiest way to take the turn is to lean yourself and the bike. To do so, push down hard on your outside pedal (this balances the bike and prevents hitting the pavement with your inside pedal) and lean with the bike as needed to negotiate the turn.

Push the bars

For quick, sharp turns, you'll need to lean the bike far down while keeping your body fairly upright. The same setup applies: Press down hard on your outside pedal. Shift your butt backward on the saddle, keep your weight low over the top tube, and press down on the handlebar with your inside hand while keeping your torso upright. As you come into the curve, press the inside knee in toward the top tube. This allows the bike to shift farther into the turn, while you stay centered over it. (For more quick cornering techniques, see "Instant Turn" in "Emergency Maneuvers," page 80.)

Quick cornering takes practice. And unfortunately, there's no way to get better at it than by doing it. Work on your technique on quiet, open roads with some safe bail-out points (i.e., you won't fly off a cliff) to take if you screw up and where you can see traffic a long way off. Whatever you do, always ride within your comfort level and don't take dumb chances. I know plenty of people who have earned an ambulance ride to the ER because they rode over their head. Unless someone is writing you checks to ride, take your time and let your skills come up to speed at your own comfort level.

CLIMBING: ASCEND LIKE AN ANGEL

Gravity sucks. That's more than a juvenile pun; it's the absolute truth, especially when you're on two wheels trying to scale a 12 percent grade. With each and every pedal stroke, you can feel the forces of physics pulling you back to Earth. It's no surprise, of course, that the best climbers tend to be wispy waifs. They have less mass to lift up the mountain. Strength helps, too, however. Strong muscles give you a good power-to-weight ratio—a fancy way of saying that a muscle-bound rugby player can still be queen of the hill because she's got the strength to literally carry her own weight. Even if you're more fluff than buff, technique goes a long way. I know quite a few fitness freaks who can't climb a hill of beans and plenty of soft-around-the-center riders who can crush the most vertical climbs. Below are some tips on how to use mind over mountain:

Relax

Here's a little experiment: Grasp this book with both hands. Now grip it *really, really* tightly, clench your teeth, drop your head, and hold on for dear life until your ears pop. Tired? Now get on a bike and mimic that same posture while pedaling uphill. You get the picture. The more energy you waste grimacing and white-knuckling the bars, the less you have to get to the top. Keep your head up, shoulders down, hands loose, and enjoy the climb. Think light, pleasant thoughts, and try to keep your feet light on the pedals. Many climbs are only as bad as you make them out to be.

Open up and let the air flow in

Climbing takes lots of energy. That means you need even more oxygen than usual to keep those fat-blasting furnaces churning. Maximize your intake by keeping your shoulders down, back straight, and chest open. Concentrate on taking deep, full breaths and maintain a loose, controlled pedaling style. And remember to pace yourself. If you try charging up the hill straight out of the gate, you'll get winded quickly, and it'll be that much harder to relax and find your rhythm.

Slide back

As a woman, your turbo chargers are located in your glutes. To tap into those turbines, slide back on the saddle. That will fully engage your glutes to generate more force over the top of the pedal stroke and help keep your heels down as you pull back around the bottom of the revolution.

Get up and go

Seated climbing is technically the most efficient because it uses fewer muscles and less energy. But there comes a time when you need to get out of the saddle to keep momentum. How often you stand is a matter of personal preference. I used to plant my butt on my saddle, rising up only when absolutely necessary. Now I prefer to dance on the pedals, alternatively getting up for a few yards and sitting down for a few.

When you feel like you need to stand, click into the next-larger gear and get up right at the top of the pedal stroke to minimize loss of momentum. Shift your hips forward, but keep most of your weight back and over the bottom bracket, where the pedal cranks connect to the bike. (Leaning too far forward puts excess weight on the front wheel, causing the back wheel to spin out and slow you down.) Gently pull on the handlebars to generate more power as you push down on the pedals—right arm pull, right foot push; left arm pull, left foot push—so the bike rocks naturally from side to side underneath you. When you're ready to sit back down, downshift and smoothly sit down at the top of a pedal stroke.

Dig in

We may not have ten-mile climbs like they do out West, but here in Pennsylvania we are walled in by short climbs so steep you almost expect to be upside down riding around a loop at the top. There are two ways to tackle these vertical assaults. One is to shift your weight *way* back, hold the top of the handlebar close to the stem, and pull back on the bar with both hands as you power through each pedal stroke. The other is to stand up and try to hold your bike as straight up as possible as you use your body weight to push the pedals down and around. The key is keeping all your energy focused on forward momentum.

You'll inevitably see some riders who "tack" up steep climbs, riding in a zigzag motion. That helps lessen the grade, because you're cutting across the hill rather than straight up. But it lengthens the climb and is more dangerous on the road because you're bobbing and weaving in front of other riders and traffic.

If all else fails, walk. Seriously. Cycling snobs may gasp and cluck their tongues at the very word. But we've all been there. Heck, I've seen fit triathletes hoofing their bikes up steep ascents during races. It doesn't feel great. But it's not the end of the world either. Just make sure you come back again (and maybe again) until you can conquer that climb.

Finish strong

When you finally reach the crest of the climb, pedal faster! Many riders slow to a crawl as they near the top because the hard work is behind them. With all your momentum gone, it's that much harder to get going again. Instead, keep pedaling, trying to pick up speed, until you feel gravity start to pull you over the other side.

DESCENDING: ALL THE REWARD WITHOUT THE RISK

Talk to any longtime cyclist about why they love to ride, and they'll inevitably turn to avian imagery: "It feels like flying." For those of us who will never pull a Cessna into the clouds, riding a bike is as close as we can come to having wings. And nowhere is that feeling keener than when you're heading downhill.

As a cyclist, descents are your reward for the work of climbing. But that reward inevitably carries some risk. The more speed you pick up, the harder it is to stop suddenly or make a quick turn. The number one rule for safe descending is to anticipate the unexpected. You obviously can't worry yourself silly about all the "what ifs." Yes, a roadside rabbit could launch itself into your front wheel and wreck your day, but you shouldn't let that slow you down. Instead, watch for bumps and debris, pay close attention to side roads and driveways where a car might come out in front of you, and consider road signs with lots of sharp turns and squiggles as a tip that you should scrub your speed. Other tips for getting down the mountain whole and happy include:

Keep your butt back

The lower your center of gravity, the more stable you'll feel. Shift your weight back and lower your body over the top tube. If you start to pick up a little too much speed, keep your butt back but sit up slightly to catch the wind with your torso, which will slow you down. Keep both feet parallel to the ground (unless you're going through a corner) to help support your weight in this position.

Brake with both hands

Hitting the front brake too hard makes the bike very difficult to handle and may even send you over the handlebars. Hitting just the back brake will cause the rear wheel to skid out but won't stop you very well. Use both evenly to slow the bike while still keeping it under control. On long descents, it's wise to periodically feather the brakes. Brake lightly to scrub speed, then release, and repeat as necessary to get down the hill without losing control.

Pull your parachute

Use your body as a human brake to slow down on long descents. Simply sit up tall and make your body big, so you catch all the wind you can (if you have a jacket on, you actually do look like a parachute from behind when you do this). You can even stand up on the pedals (but keep your weight back) to increase the resistance. It's an easy way to slow down without braking.

Use a high gear

Depending on the pitch of the descent, you may need to pedal, or you might choose to coast all the way down. Either way, use a high gear. A little tension in the chain helps you control the bike.

BRAKING: SMOOTH SLOWING AND STOPPING

Your brakes stop the bike. Obviously a good thing. But, as with ice cream and coconut cream pie, you can definitely have too much of a good thing—and that's very often the case with newbie cyclists and their brakes. You don't want to be careening out of control, but don't be afraid of carrying a little speed either. As you know if you've ever tried to ride *really* slowly, your bike is more stable when it's rolling briskly. When you slam on the brakes, it becomes very unstable very quickly, and you're more likely to crash. Some cardinal rules of braking:

Two fingers is all it takes

The only time you *may* need a full grip on your brakes is when you're making an emergency stop suddenly to avoid a collision. Otherwise, keep most of your fingers wrapped around the bars and use just your index finger, or your index and middle fingers, to work the brake lever. In this position, you have maximum control of your bike and are less likely to brake too hard. If you can't reach or it's too difficult to pull the lever with just one or two fingers, ask your bike shop about short-reach levers, which are made for smaller hands.

Shift back

When you hit the brakes, your bike slows down but your body keeps going, sending your weight forward over the front wheel and making it difficult to steer. Counter this effect by shifting your weight back on the saddle as you brake.

Easy on the front

Up to 70 percent of your braking power comes from the front brake. Use it with a light touch.

Brake more when wet

You know from driving a car that it takes longer to stop on wet roads: It's even worse with a bike because your rims are less grippy when they're wet, so your brakes don't work as well. During long descents on wet roads, keep your brakes ever so slightly squeezed. This helps keep them free from excess water to allow for quicker stopping. (For more on braking in special situations, see "Emergency Maneuvers," page 79.)

DRINKING PROBLEMS

Some skills that experienced cyclists take completely for granted are the most daunting to novices. Getting a drink is one of those skills. A friend of mine did her first triathlon in a severely dehydrated state because she was too scared to reach for her water bottle at high speed (and too competitive to slow down and drink!). When you need to ride one-handed for any reason, first place your hands on the top of the bars close to the stem in the center of the handlebar. This is the easiest way to keep the bike centered and steady and will keep you from veering unexpectedly if you hit a bump. When getting a drink, glance at the bottle cage area only briefly when pulling out the bottle and again when replacing it. The more you do it, the more automatic it becomes, until you won't even need to look down to drink on the fly.

PACK RIDING: FOLLOW THE LEADER . . .

Cycling is like dancing. It's fun to shake and shimmy in the privacy of your living room, but it's more fun with a crowd. As in dancing, there are also a few steps to follow so you don't step on anyone's toes.

How rigid the rules are depends on the pack. Some groups are pretty rigid; they roll in an organized paceline (where all riders form

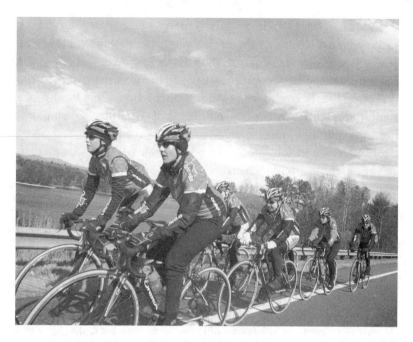

Riding in a paceline is the best way to cover miles. When you're up front, share the work and enjoy the view—then roll to the back to recover and enjoy the ride.
Photo courtesy of Team Cheerwine

a tight single-file line, taking turns pulling at the front and fighting the wind) or a double paceline and expect riders to fall in line. Other packs are pretty loose, falling into a line when it makes sense, breaking up and chitchatting when space allows.

At its best, paceline riding is a transcendent experience. The group can ride faster with less effort than any single rider can alone. And it literally feels like poetry in motion as the group follows the rhythms of the road.

At its worst, paceline riding is a killjoy. I've been in many a paceline that disintegrates into a Darwinian survival of the fittest with guys ratcheting up the pace every time they take the lead and dropping riders off the back like so much litter.

Your best bet is finding a mixed group where there are riders of varying fitness levels and the pack makes a point of not leaving anyone behind. Ask your local bike shop if they know a casual group you can join. You can also try practicing with a friend or two. All you need is a wheel to follow, and you have a mini-paceline. As soon as you're comfortable with your basic bike riding skills (shifting, stopping, riding a straight line), you're ready to practice a paceline.

Once you find your group, the number one rule is to ride predictably. Even if the group is casual, it's important that the riders around you can anticipate your actions. That means riding in a straight line, keeping a fairly steady pace, and not making any sudden stops or swerves without alerting the rest of the riders. When riding in a paceline:

Get in close

The main purpose of a paceline is to get the benefits of drafting. Scientists have found that you use 30% less effort drafting than you do riding solo. But I'm here to tell you, sometimes it's almost 100% less effort. When I get behind my 6'2", 185-pound husband and his friends, I feel like I could sit up and order a pizza. I barely have to work. But you never get this magical feeling if you don't get in close, which can be scary the first few times. Ideally, you want to be just about a foot (or less if you're *really* comfortable) away from their back wheel. But don't start there. Begin by riding about one bike length behind someone. As you get more comfortable, gradually close the gap. You may also feel more comfortable riding a few inches to one side or the other of the wheel in front of you, as that will give you a little more reaction time, should that rider do something unpredictable. Once you get about a wheel length away from the rider in front of you, you'll start to enjoy the benefits of drafting.

Pull off, pull through

When the rider at the front is ready for a break, she checks back for oncoming cars, drifts to the left and allows the pack to pull forward, then drifts back, taking her place at the end of the train. Sometimes it's helpful to point left as you're ready to pull off so the rider behind you is fully aware of your intentions.

Keep the pace

Sounds obvious, but try to maintain the same pace as the pack. This is especially important when you take your turn up front. Too often the rider taking the lead charges ahead and the pack splinters as the pace increases. Sometimes this charge is an ego-driven exercise ("Look how fast *I* can pull!). But often it's just an innocent mistake. You feel fresh because you haven't been working that hard in the back and you don't want to be the one to slow production, so you turn on the gas.

If you have a computer on your bike monitoring your speed, it's easy to just check the speed periodically and try to keep the same pace when you're in front. If not, just be conscious not to accelerate when you take the lead. When you're in the midst of the paceline, avoid braking. Instead ease up on your pedaling effort (this is called soft pedaling) to slow down or drift ever so slightly to the left to catch some wind and scrub your speed.

Take short pulls

Don't feel like you have to sit up there and pull everyone along for thirty miles. Pacelines work best when the lead riders limit themselves to half-mile pulls because it keeps everyone fresh.

Watch your front wheel

Do not overlap your front wheel with the back wheel of the bike you're following. If that rider has to swerve suddenly and hits you, you'll be the one to hit the pavement when she taps into you.

Call out cars and other hazards

Communication is key to safe, happy group riding. The riders in front call out such oncoming hazards as potholes, gravel, roadkill, cars pulling out of driveways, and so on by pointing down and calling out "Gravel!" or "Squirrel!" etc. They should also call out turns and stop signs well in advance so the pack can prepare. The caboose in the back alerts the pack to approaching cars (unless, of course, you're on a heavily trafficked road) by calling out "Car back!" Everyone is responsible for keeping the pack together. If you see someone falling back, call "Sit up" or "Slow down a little."

If you get a flat tire or develop another problem that forces you to stop quickly, don't panic. Just yell out "Stopping!" and try to keep your forward momentum as best you can as the other riders scurry around you.

Keep your eyes up

The cyclist in front of you might have cute buns, but staring directly at them as you ride ahead is risky business. (It also makes you miss all the pretty scenery.) Ditto for staring at the wheel ahead of you. Lift your eyes and gaze down the road, so you can see what's coming. Glance down occasionally.

Climb with care

It's hard to keep a paceline together when the road tilts up. It's wise to give the rider in front of you a little more space when climbing; they may slow down or stand up. Standing is particularly troublesome, because there's a tendency for your bike to drift back (and potentially into the wheel behind you) when you stand. If you do need to get out of the saddle and you're in a close group, announce "Standing!" before you get up.

Leave room on descents

Pacelines often spread out or completely break apart down hills, especially if they're steep, because gravity takes over and larger riders will naturally descend more quickly (and enjoy the thrill of doing so). On gradual descents you can stay close.

Eat and drink in the back

Save your drinking, eating, and nose blowing for the back of the line, where your sudden movements won't disrupt the flow of motion.

Do the double

If your group is large (say, more than four or five riders), it makes sense to double up and ride two-by-two in a double paceline. Different rules apply depending on the group. Sometimes the echelon is in constant rotation, with one line moving faster than the other. So if you are the front rider on the inside, you would drift left (remaining in front) but then drift back, and the next front rider comes right to left. This is pretty tricky to pull off. The easier technique is for the front riders to both pull to the outside and the pack to pull through, allowing them to drift back.

EMERGENCY MANEUVERS: DON'T LEAVE HOME WITHOUT THEM

Emergency maneuvers should really be called "evasive" maneuvers, because that's what they really are—tricks of physics that help you avoid what seems inevitable: a nasty crash. When I became a League Cycling Instructor (or LCI, as the League of American Bicyclists likes to call us), we spent the better part of a day in a parking lot dotted with small orange cones and sawed-off tennis balls practicing these butt-saving skills until they were branded on our brains.

I'll admit, after an hour, I was a little like an antsy sophomore suffering through algebra II, muttering, "When am I going to use this?" But, sure enough, on a mountain bike ride months later I was speeding down a slip of single-track trail when without warning (funny how there are no road signs in the wilderness . . .) the trail disappeared, banging a hard left along a ridge. Dead ahead was nothing but blue sky above and rocks below. Guess who was happy for her emergency maneuvers? I pulled a picture-perfect "instant turn" and avoided sure disaster. Many of these are fun to practice in parking lots as you're waiting for your friends to show up for your Sunday ride.

EMERGENCY STOP

Say you're buzzing down the road minding your own business and a kid in a Domino's hat flings open his car door right in your path. You can pray that double order of cheesy breadsticks softens the blow, or you can pull an emergency stop. Place both feet parallel to the ground, lift your butt, and shift your weight way back behind the saddle; extend your arms and sink your weight low, dropping your torso toward the top tube. Then give your brakes a tight squeeze. Do this all in one smooth move, so it almost looks like you're trying to throw your bike forward and your body back. This is one you should be sure to practice; you never know when you might need it.

INSTANT TURN

This emergency maneuver is useful whenever you have to make a super quick turn, whether it's to avoid careening off a cliff at an unexpected hairpin (as above) or to avert a car that makes an unannounced turn right in front of you. To do it, pedal straight ahead at a moderate speed. Now imagine that a car just turned right directly in front of you and you're heading right for it. Initiate the turn by flicking your wrists to snap the bars slightly left, the *opposite* direction you want to go in. This snap forces you into a rapid right-direction lean. Then immediately turn right, into the lean. Like magic! It works every time. Once you master it, this is also an outstanding technique for ripping through tight corners at speed.

ROCK DODGE

The roadsides are filled with an amazing array of obstacles: broken bottles, dead animals, chunks of concrete. Most often you have plenty of time to change your line of travel to avoid these hazards. But sometimes they come up quick. When they do, you can avoid them seamlessly with almost no disruption in momentum by pulling a rock dodge. Keep pedaling straight toward the obstacle until you are just a few inches from it. Immediately steer left, then right, then straighten your handlebars and roll on. The first turn gets your front tire around the obstacle and throws you into a lean. The immediate countersteer corrects your balance, tracking your back tire around and right back in line. Both tires evade the bump and continue a straight path at speed. This is a good one to practice with something, like a sawed-off tennis ball, that won't buck you off your bike should you actually hit it.

BUNNY HOP

This classic mountain bike maneuver can come in handy on the road should you encounter a large divot, sharp lip, or other unavoidable obstacle in your path. As the name implies, you simply lift your bike up in the air and leap over it. It takes some practice, but it's easier than it sounds. Start by standing on your pedals and crouching like a cat on your bike. Your elbows, knees, and hips should be bent with your weight sinking downward as though you were loading your arms and legs like springs. As you approach the obstacle (you have to time it pretty close), explode straight upward, pulling on the handlebars and twisting your wrists forward to help bring the rear wheel up and over. *Keep your hands off the brakes.* Land with your elbows and knees soft on the other side. Sit down and continue on your way. This one takes practice; be sure to practice over something like a jump rope or a stretched-out spare tube that won't knock you off your bike if you don't clear it.

CANINE EVASION

Dogs love bikes. Friendly little Benji dogs dash in hyper-speed bliss straight toward their spokes. Killer Cujo types relish the personal challenge: "I couldn't catch that Hummer, but that one on those little wheels is all mine!" Surprisingly, most dogs listen if you yell at them. A loud authoritative "Go home!" usually startles them enough to give you time to hustle out of their range. If that doesn't work (and there will be a time when it doesn't), grab your water bottle and spray the dog in the face. It slows them down just enough for you to make a quick getaway. If the dog is close and menacing, stop, place your bike between you and the dog, and wait for the owner to get it under control.

PUSHING AND FALLING

Track riders and serious road racers compete in very close quarters with many cyclists vying for the same piece of pavement. To prepare for these conditions, many will actually practice pushing drills, where they ride side-by-side on a grassy field and nudge each other with elbows, give shoves, and otherwise turn cycling into a contact sport. It's actually fun to do, and you'll likely be surprised at how well your bike stays up even when someone tries to bump you over. It's a great skill to have even if you never plan to set wheel on a racecourse, because it increases your stability and bike handling skills. Just start gently!

It's also a good idea to know how to fall, though I don't generally advise practicing it (though some riders do). Just try to remember a few basic rules. One is to avoid sticking your arm out to break your fall, unless it's a very controlled situation and you're going over slowly. It's a natural instinct, but it's the surest way to break your wrist or collarbone. Instead, tuck your chin to your chest and roll onto your shoulder. This distributes the impact over a broader area and minimizes the chance for injury.

IDIOT AVOIDANCE

People sometimes ask if I'm afraid to ride by myself, being a woman and all. The short answer is no. I know bad things happen. I know there are bad people. But I'm just as likely to meet them in a mall parking lot (maybe more so?) than on my bike on a Sunday morning. In the twenty-plus years I've been riding, I've had very few unpleasant encounters with motorists or pedestrians (and these inevitably occurred when I was out with a large group, which tend to aggravate motorists a little more than a solitary cyclist). I have friends who have ridden across entire states by themselves and say the same.

Sure, I've gotten a few whistles or woo-hoos, but even those are infrequent. Mostly, when someone yells something out the window to me, it's encouragement, which is cool. Still, I do try to play it smart. I tell my husband where I'm going and about how long I'll be. I carry my cell phone and some cash. If I'm going to be more remote than I feel comfortable with, I'll also carry pepper spray (it also makes me feel safer should I encounter an unfriendly canine). I also never ride with my iPod, so I'm aware of my surroundings. If you're very concerned, ride with a friend or stick to more populated areas.

RULES OF THE ROAD

The law says bikes have the same rights to the roads as cars do. That means we also have the same responsibilities. I'll be the first to admit, I'm no saint. I'm sure to sail through a lonely stop sign on a quiet Saturday afternoon when I can see no one around for a country mile. But I play it straight when I'm in traffic, and I refuse to ride in packs that cavalierly ignore traffic signs and anger motorists by crying that they belong on the roads yet refuse to obey the rules of the road. They're dangerous and give our sport a bad name. If we're to coexist with 2,000-pound vehicles, we should play fair and square. Here's how:

RIDE RIGHT

Riding on the wrong side of the road is a leading cause of cycling accidents. It may seem like a good idea to ride on the left where you can see cars coming, but it's super dangerous for reasons you learned in eighth-grade math. If you're traveling 15 MPH and a truck is coming your way at 40 MPH, combined you are approaching each other at 55 MPH—head-on. That leaves little reaction time for you or the truck driver should your paths come too close. Turn yourself around in the same scenario and the truck is approaching you just 25 MPH faster. The driver has much more time to spot you, slow down, and maneuver around you. The driver also expects to see other traffic traveling in his or her direction. No one expects to see traffic coming at them in their own lane. Remember, being struck from behind makes up a *very* small percentage of bike accidents. If you ride predictably and responsibly, cars can accommodate you.

BUT NOT TOO FAR RIGHT . . .

Cycling experts and advocates have argued for years about how far right cyclists should ride. Some will contend you should ride as far right as possible, while others argue you should always "take the lane" (ride farther left with the flow of traffic), so cars are forced to slow down and pass you safely rather than squeezing by you and maybe forcing you off the road. I'm a big fan of playing it both ways. If there's a nice wide, clean, clear shoulder, I use it. If the shoulder's a mess or the road is very narrow and I don't want cars squeaking by me at an unsafe distance, I move farther out into the lane, so they're forced to make a clear, safe pass.

Commuters who frequently ride city streets should blend into traffic as much as possible. Ride a couple of feet left of parked cars to minimize your risk of getting doored should someone open their car door into your path (also make a habit of glancing into the side-view mirrors of cars as you pass to spot motorists who might be ready to step out of their vehicles). Don't weave in and out of the parking lane. For cars to see you and respond to you, you need to be visible and predictable at all times.

USE YOUR SIGNALS

Let motorists know what you're doing. If you're turning left, extend your left arm and point left. Turning right? Do the same thing, only in that direction. Yes, I know that technically a right-turn signal is done with a bent left arm, but don't expect sixteen-year-old Emily cruising and chatting behind you in her mom's Beemer to have a clue what you're doing with your arm jutting up in the air. Everyone understands what pointing means. When you're stopping, just extend your left arm down at a diagonal with your palm facing back.

SEE AND BE SEEN

The farther out motorists can see you, the safer you are. Wear bright colors. If you ride at dusk, dawn, or in the dark, *always* use a front headlight and a red rear light (preferably blinking, which makes you more noticeable). Commuters who spend a lot of time riding in the twilight hours should invest in reflective clothing. You can buy entire cycling outfits (jerseys, arm warmers, tights) made with illumiNITE fabric that lights up like a Christmas tree when headlights hit it.

BEWARE DANGER ZONES

There are some surfaces that are inherently dangerous and require special attention. Watch for:

Railroad tracks

These are always a menace. Try to cross as close to perpendicular as possible (with your tire approaching the tracks at a 90-degree angle). Be careful but don't go super slow. It's easier to cross when you're carrying a little speed.

Sewer grates and manhole covers

These are sunken into the road, made of metal, and often have bumps, grooves, and other tire catching features. Ditto for metal grate bridges. They're *very* slippery when wet. Avoid them—especially sewer grates—when possible. If you have to cross metal grate bridges, ride a straight and steady line over them. And stay loose. Tensing up makes you more likely to crash.

Road markings

Painted pavement is also slippery when wet, so avoid crossing over it in rainy conditions.

TAKE A LOOK BACK

Scanning behind you for traffic is an essential skill for road riding. Some riders like using "third eyes" (little rearview mirrors that extend from their helmet) but most don't. Statistically, very few bike accidents are the result of getting hit from behind. Most happen in front of you, which is where your attention needs to be. Mirrors can be a distraction from that. But you *do* have to look back from time to time, especially when you're turning or changing lanes. The danger is swerving into an oncoming car as you look back to check for traffic; you'll notice that as you look over your shoulder, you lean a little, which causes your bike to turn in that direction. To avoid this common mishap, practice keeping your shoulders squared and applying slightly more pressure to the right hand as you briefly glance back over your left shoulder. You can practice on quiet roads. Try to stay on the white line while scanning back. Your bike shouldn't veer more than an inch or so off the line.

PLAY NICE

Put yourself in the motorists' bucket seats and try to ride courteously and make life easy for them. If you're riding with others on a heavily trafficked road, get in a single file. If riding side-by-side on a quiet country road, scoot over to let the occasional car go by. Wave at cars and show your appreciation if you've held them up. Don't cruise all the way to the front of a long line of traffic at a stoplight, forcing cars to pass you again if they had a hard time getting around you the first time. Finally, no matter how mad someone makes you, don't shake your fist, flip them off, or shout unseemly things. That's a battle you always lose.

OFF-ROAD BASICS

Mountain biking is like skiing—it's best learned in baby steps. Just as you wouldn't dream of stepping off the ski lift onto a black diamond slope for your first ever run down the mountain, you shouldn't expect to take your maiden mountain bike voyage on highly technical (e.g., rocky, steep, log-strewn) terrain.

First, get the feeling for off-road riding on a nearby bridal trail or cinder path. As you become more comfortable, venture onto some rougher terrain like rocky or wooded single track (a hiking-type trail usually strewn with rocks, roots, and water crossings). Though mountain biking is best learned by doing (and watching other more skilled riders), starting with some basic skill knowledge helps. Here are a few off-road essentials:

LOOK WHERE YOU WANT TO GO

There are lots of things on the trail—pointy rocks, ditches, off-camber roots, to name a few—that you don't want to hit. By all means, don't lock your eyes on them. Your bike has this uncanny knack for going in the direction you're looking. So the first rule of off-road riding is to keep your eyes on the path you want to take, fixing your gaze well ahead of what is immediately in front of your tire. Mountain bikers call this desirable path of least resistance "the line." The more you ride, the better you'll be able to pick your lines and ride smoothly around and through obstacles of all kinds.

KEEP YOUR BUTT BACK

One of the worst crashes mountain bikers face is the "endo," short for "end over end," a forward roll over your front tire with you ending up flat on your back. One of the most common causes of endos is pitching your weight too far forward while going downhill, especially if you're also using the front brake. When traveling down a steep descent, it's essential that you shift your weight back to maintain your center of gravity between your wheels. On very steep pitches, you may need to put your butt all the way off and behind the saddle. That way even if you have to hit the brakes to scrub speed or your front tire hits a rock or root, your back end will stay firmly grounded. You'll be amazed at the steep pitches you can sail down with ease by simply shifting your weight in this way.

GIVE YOUR WHEELS ROOM TO WORK

Mountain bikes are designed with fat tires and shock absorbers that allow you to roll over small to mid-size obstacles on the trail. It's your job to "unweight" your tires to help it along. Be conscious of not leaning too heavily on your handlebars. Instead, keep your weight evenly distributed between your hands, feet, and butt. As you approach an obstacle on the trail, press down on the bars to compress the shock absorber (this will help you raise the front wheel), then lift up on the bars to pull the front tire up and over whatever is in the way. After your front tire clears the obstacle, lift your butt off the saddle to unweight your back tire so it can clear it as well.

GIVE YOUR WHEELS WEIGHT TO WORK

On the flip side, sometimes you need to put more weight on your tires to help them do their job. This is especially true when you're climbing. To make it up a steep hill, you need traction, especially in the back wheel. To help the back tire dig in, shift your weight back slightly. If the hill is so steep that your front tire starts lifting off the ground, lean forward to put more weight toward the front, then pull straight back on the handlebars as you climb. For very steep pitches, you may need to hover your butt off the saddle and crouch over the bike to use your whole body to power the pedals, while maintaining maximum traction.

MOMENTUM IS YOUR FRIEND

Remember high school physics? A body in motion wants to stay in motion unless acted on by an outside force. Your bike wants to continue rolling in the direction you're traveling, and mountain bikes are designed to roll over rough terrain. You'll be far more stable over small rocks and roots if you're carrying a little speed (because you have more momentum) than if you're crawling along getting bumped off course by every little obstacle in the path.

USE THE FORCE

If you err on the side of easier gears on your road bike, try using a slightly higher one on the mountain. Though you still want to maintain a comfortable, efficient pedaling cadence (as opposed to mashing down on your pedals), you'll find that it's easier to literally spin your wheels on the sketchy dirt and slippery mud that you'll find off-road. By using a slightly harder gear, you can get more torque to power the bike through more difficult terrain.

RIDE RELAXED

The first time you ride through a rock-strewn path, you may have the urge to tense up and try to control your bike as it hops and jumps through the bumpy terrain. That kind of strong-arming only serves to make the ride rougher, because you're not allowing the bike to ebb and flow naturally. Instead, relax your body and keep your elbows and knees slightly bent at all times, so the bike has room to move beneath you as you gently guide it down the trail.

DON'T GO OUT THERE ALONE

It's one thing to ride your local rail trail or park paths by yourself. It's quite another to go way off-road by your lonesome. I know women who do it, but I'm not one and I don't recommend it. Not just because you're a woman (though we all know we have special risks because we are) but because unpredictable things can happen on mountain bikes—you hit a rock you didn't see, a stick flies into your spokes and sends you over your handlebars—and if you're on some remote trail, it can be impossible to find help, even with a cell phone. Ride with friends. It's safer and more fun.

A STUDENT FOR LIFE

Learning to ride is a lifelong process. And sometimes you have to stop and weigh the benefits with the risks. One of my favorite riding friends is molasses sweet and slow on descents because they scare her. One spring she decided she'd take more risks, and she ended up crashing on a tight corner. She's since gone back to her leisurely descending ways, and that's just fine. She'd rather spend time riding than rehabbing. On the flip side, my favorite mountain biking girlfriend is always pushing the envelope. She studies descents, asks other riders tons of questions about their techniques, and goes for it. She's had her fair share of wrecks, but, to her, mastering a skill is worth the spill. There's no right or wrong—just what works for you.

5

How to Train

A Little Structure Goes a Long Way

When I first started racing, I did what most women do. I rode my bike . . . a lot. In my mind, the more miles I put in, the faster I should get. It didn't work out so well. I ended up more fatigued than fit, and a lot crabbier, but not much faster. Then I got smart. I put together a week-by-week plan that included structured intervals, true rest days, and concrete goals. It was like having a magic wand! (Not really, but it worked nearly as well.) I racked up some of the best races of my life. More important, I felt fit, happy, and insanely energetic.

When riding has become an essential part of your life, you should think about training, even if you have no intention of racing. Adding a little structure to your regular riding routine can help you reach all kinds of goals, including losing weight or finishing your next charity ride feeling fresh or finally beating your friends up your toughest hometown climb.

Training is also motivating. You're less likely to skip riding if you have a specific workout on your calendar. The miles fly by when you have a mission. And it's just plain fun to feel fast. Here, then, are the essentials of training and how they can work for you:

HOW TRAINING WORKS

Every pedal stroke you take is a form of training. Your body registers that you're cranking out a certain level of effort, and it starts adapting so it's sure to be ready if you want to do it again. That is all training is—adaptation. The more specifically you train, the more specifically your body adapts to what you want to do.

In cycling, the biggest adaptation your body makes is how well it uses oxygen. The first time you go out for a ride, you'll probably find yourself huffing and puffing up every little hill. Over time, the hill gets easier, until after a few weeks, you're barely out of breath. Here's what happens:

YOUR HEART GETS STRONGER

Your heart is a muscle that acts like a pump to send oxygen-rich blood through your body. When you ride, especially if you're working hard, your heart gets stronger so it can squeeze out more blood with every beat. That means it doesn't have to beat as fast or work as hard to help you get up hills or sprint down the road. You'll notice this both on and off the bike. It's common for a new rider to see their resting heart rate (how many times your heart beats per minute when you're just sitting around) drop 10 or 15 beats as they get more fit. While sedentary women have heart rates approaching 70 or 80 BPM (beats per minute), their cycling sisters usually hum along at just 50 or 60 BPM.

THE CAPILLARY NETWORK GROWS

Your legs need all the oxygen-rich blood they can get to fuel your cells' aerobic energy-making engines. As you get more fit, your cardiovascular system literally forges hundreds of new capillaries into your muscles to maximize circulation.

AEROBIC ENZYMES INCREASE

Your body produces more aerobic enzymes so it can extract more oxygen from your blood to burn fat and make energy. The better you are at burning fat, the longer you can ride without hitting the wall.

YOU RAISE YOUR "ROOF"

As you'll see later in this chapter, your body has an endurance ceiling, called lactate threshold. That's the point at which your muscles literally scream "Slow down!" because they're burning so much (though scientists now know it's not the lactic acid actually doing the burning; rather, the body is in a state of acidosis due to proton production). With training, you can raise this ceiling, so you can ride faster and farther before your muscles slam on the brakes.

Any type of regular riding will help you achieve these goals, but structured training will help you achieve them more quickly and efficiently. More important, a training plan will help you shape up without burning out.

DO YOU NEED TO SEE A DOC?

Most healthy women don't need to see a doctor before they start training. That's especially true if you've been riding or otherwise exercising for a while already. But it's important to take the necessary precautions and see a physician first if you have health problems. If you have an existing heart condition, chest pain, dizzy spells, or other potentially dangerous symptoms, get your doc's stamp of approval before you embark on a training program.

MEASURING YOUR EFFORT

The single most important element behind any training plan is knowing how hard you're working at any given time during a ride. If you're supposed to ride hard, you need to know how hard; likewise, when it's time to go easy, you need to know how much to back off. There are a few ways to measure intensity:

USE YOUR HEAD—RPE

One of the simplest tools for measuring your effort is called "rating of perceived exertion" (RPE). It's a techie way of saying: On a scale of 1 to 10, how hard are you working?

Devised by exercise scientists to measure intensity of exercise, RPE simply assigns numbers to your efforts. The lowest rating, 1, is coasting down a long lazy country road while barely putting any pressure on the pedals; 10 is sprinting up a mountainside away from a pack of hungry wolves. You judge how hard you're riding by placing your effort on a scale between those two extremes.

Perceived exertion is free (you don't have to buy any fancy equipment). And it works; studies pitting RPE against pricey training tools found that RPE works just as well when used properly. That "when used properly" part is essential. The problem with RPE is that it's easy to ignore. Without a concrete indicator of your efforts, such as a number on a screen, it's easy to push yourself too hard during recovery and not dig deep enough during hard work intervals.

One way to keep yourself honest is monitoring your breathing—a favorite method of a colleague of mine who trains athletes of all levels. "Nothing gives you an instant and honest evaluation of your effort like your breathing," says James Herrera, owner of Performance Driven Coaching in Colorado Springs. He recommends following this scale:

Zone 1
Deep, steady, relaxed breathing. That's your aerobic, endurance training zone. It's an RPE of 3 to 5.

Zone 2

Short, quick, rhythmic breathing. That's your lactate threshold zone. It's an RPE of about 6 to 8.

Zone 3

Gasping your lungs inside out. That's your VO2 max training zone. It's an RPE of 9 to 10.

If you choose to judge your intensity using RPE, keeping a close check on which breathing zone you're in will help you stay on target. The advantage of using breathing zones is obvious: You're always breathing, so you always have something to gauge your efforts. It's completely free and easy to use. The disadvantage is that the training zones are very broad. With more sensitive monitoring systems (like heart rate, explained below), you can break down your training zones further to fine-tune your efforts.

LACTIC ACID IS NOT THE ENEMY

Lactic acid is probably the most wrongly maligned metabolic process in the history of human activity. For nearly a century (starting with experiments in the 1920s), exercise scientists have blamed lactic acid—a by-product of burning carbohydrates during hard exercise—on the muscle burn and fatigue that forces you to slow down during high-intensity exercise,

Well, guess what? They were wrong all along. Today we know that the body actually produces lactic acid as a supplemental fuel, and the more you train, the better you get at using lactic acid for energy. It works like this: During hard exercise, your muscles convert some of your stored carbs (glycogen) to lactic acid. That lactic acid is taken into the cells' mitochondria (their furnace) and used as fuel to make energy. In untrained people, muscle cell mitochondria aren't all that big, so they can't take in as much lactic acid, and they shut down the system (fatigue) faster. Training increases the mass of your mitochondria, so seasoned cyclists can burn more lactic acid and work harder longer.

This understanding of lactic acid is nothing short of a sea change in exercise science, so don't be surprised if you still hear otherwise sharp trainers trash-talking lactic acid as if it's the enemy. They just haven't caught up to the science.

LISTEN TO YOUR HEART

Your heart is like your body's electric meter. Just as watching how fast the dial spins tells you how much energy you're using as you turn on the lights and run the hair dryer, recording how many times your heart beats per minute tells you how hard your body is working as you're riding down the road.

For many years, heart rate monitoring was the gold standard for measuring training intensity. Though serious racers now measure their power output as well (see "The Power of Watts," page 99), heart rate remains an important training tool. Here's how it works:

Tune in

First and foremost you need a heart rate monitor. A heart rate monitor is a two-part device. The first part is a transmitter that sits on your breastbone right over your heart and stays put with a strap that wraps around your torso at the bra line. It's not as uncomfortable as it sounds, but it does take a little getting used to. The second component is a computer (similar to an odometer) that mounts to your handlebars like a cardiovascular dashboard. The sensor on your chest picks up the electrical signal from your beating heart and wirelessly transmits that information to the computer in beats per minute (BPM). Most models also let you program your training zones, and the computer beeps at you if you fall below or push above your target training zone.

Polar is the biggest name in heart rate monitors, and the company has an enormous selection to choose from. On the higher end of the price scale, you can get a heart rate monitor/cycling computer, which allows you to measure speed, distance, time, calories burned, and more along with your heart rate. If you already have a cycling computer, you can get an inexpensive, very basic monitor that comes with a watch that shows your heart rate display. (I should note that some people find that too many computers—heart rate, odometer, etc.—can interfere with each other, so sometimes it is best to consolidate in one unit for accuracy as well as simplicity.)

Max out

Heart rate training is based on your maximum heart rate (MHR)—the highest number of beats your heart can thump in one minute. So before you start, you need to figure out your max. You may have heard the old formula: 220−your age=max heart rate (which might still be used in the manual of your heart rate monitor). That formula is okay, but exercise scientists find that it underestimates MHR for older riders and overestimates it for younger riders.

A better formula: 208−0.7(your age). So for a 50-year-old woman, it would be 208−35=173 MHR. That's three beats higher than you would get using the old formula.

You can also test your maximum heart rate the old-fashioned way: Go out and push your heart rate to the max and see what you get. The obligatory caution here is that if you have any reason at all to question the safety of this level of exertion—you're older than 50, you have a strong family (or personal) history of heart problems, you've been sedentary, you're overweight, or you have any of the risk factors in the "Do You Need to See a Doc?" box on page 93—you should definitely talk to your doctor before trying this.

Warm up for 15 to 20 minutes on an indoor trainer (you can do this outside, but I think it's safer inside). Then, while maintaining a cadence of 90 to 100 RPM, increase the resistance every 30 seconds until you can't hang on any longer. Really push it those final 10 seconds as though you're gunning for Olympic gold (it helps to have a friend shouting encouragement). The highest heart rate number you hit at the end is your max. Fortunately, most heart rate monitors record and save your max heart rate, so you don't have to worry about missing it if you happen to do this test outdoors and you're watching the road instead of the monitor.

Hone your zones

After you determine your max, break your heart rate down into training zones to accomplish goals including endurance training, lactate threshold training, and recovery. Calculate your zones based on your max heart rate. For instance, a recovery heart rate for the 50-year-old woman with an MHR of 173 mentioned above would be <110 BPM ($173 \times 0.64 = 110$). The following are typical training zones coaches use:

TRAINING ZONES	
Training Zone	**% MHR**
Zone 1: recovery, easy day	60 to 64%
Zone 2: cruising, aerobic endurance	65 to 74%
Zone 3: high-level, steady aerobic ("tempo")	75 to 84%
Zone 4: lactate threshold (brisk race pace)	85 to 94%
Zone 5: max effort	95 to 100%

Though it looks extremely precise, heart rate training is somewhat of an inexact science. Pick up three different books and you'll likely find three different training zone charts with slight variations in where they draw the lines from one zone to the next. There's also a lot of individual variation. While fit riders tend to hit lactate threshold around 85% of their MHR, newbie riders may hit their ceiling at

75%. The goal of heart rate training is to be able to ride faster at the same (or even lower) heart rate.

Though heart rate is a good indicator of how hard your body is working, it's also somewhat fickle. All kinds of internal and external factors, from the weather to menstruation, can drive it up or down a few beats. It's also not always a perfect indicator of performance. For instance, you may set out to do four 30-second efforts at 90% of your max heart rate to work on your sprint performance, but if you stayed up too late watching *Sex and the City* reruns, you can get your heart rate up high without working that hard simply because you started out tired. In those cases, it can be counterproductive to simply train by the numbers.

For the best results use heart rate with RPE . . . and common sense. If you're riding at what should be an easy heart rate but you feel like you're hovering at the high end of the RPE scale, your body is telling you it needs more recovery. Listen to it.

THE POWER OF WATTS

The current state of the art in training technology is power monitoring. By definition, power (measured in watts) is the rate at which you perform work. Each time you push your pedals to roll your bike down the road against the forces of friction and gravity, you're performing work. A power meter—a device that measures pedaling force—tells you precisely how much.

The best part about power monitoring is, watts don't lie. Unlike heart rate, which can drift up and down depending on your health or how many latte grandes you've had that day, watts are always exact. They also indicate progress (or lack thereof) unequivocally. If you ride your regular loop and average 160 watts where before you could only average 120, you have clearly gotten stronger. Many riders use power meters in conjunction with heart rate to get a crystal-clear picture of their fitness and progression.

Like heart rate training, you train with a power meter by setting up power-based training zones. Most coaches base their power training zones on lactate threshold power (LTP)—the wattage you can sustain for about an hour. This number is usually about 40 watts below your max.

A favorite test for determining LTP is a 20-minute time trial. It's easiest to do this on an indoor trainer because you don't have to worry about traffic or stop signs slowing you down. Otherwise, try to find an open, relatively flat loop. Prepare by warming up for 20 minutes. Then ride hard (at about an 8 on the RPE scale) for 5 minutes. Ride easy again for 5 to 10 minutes, and you're ready to begin. Start strong (but not with a sprint), ramping up your intensity over the first minute or so, and ride for 20 minutes at the highest power you can maintain. Reduce that number by 5% and that's your LTP.

Another simple way to determine LTP is to take your average watts during a long climb. Most people climb right at their threshold. Here's a snapshot of what power ranges look like (in watts) for women of varying fitness levels.

POWER RANGES (WATTS)			
Zone	Beginner	Intermediate	Advanced
Easy, recovery	50–75	60–90	75–100
Aerobic, cruising	120–140	140–160	150–190
High-level, steady aerobic ("tempo")	140–150	160–170	190–200
Lactate threshold (brisk race pace)	155–170	175–190	205–220
VO2 max	190–240	220–280	255–280
Courtesy of James Herrera, owner of Performance Driven Coaching, Colorado Springs, www.pushyourlimit.com			

The biggest downside to power training is expense. Power meters are *pricey*, with "cheap" models coming in at more than $700. They're also complicated to install. They work by using a sensor placed at your cranks or wheel hub (in which case you need a special wheel), which transmits the data through small sensors and wires (to date, only one wireless model exists, and it's too new to comment on its performance or reliability) to a handlebar-mounted computer. They need to be properly installed and calibrated, which is more than many recreational cyclists can handle. In short, it's a great tool but a big investment.

BEWARE THE "FAT-BURNING" ZONE

This one cannot die soon enough. It all started about fifteen years ago when exercise scientists discovered that during low-intensity aerobic exercise, you burn mostly stored fat rather than carbohydrates for fuel. Aerobics instructors took off with it and created entire classes designed to keep your heart rate from getting too high and thus out of your "fat-burning zone."

Here's the real deal. Your body *does* use different sources of fuel during varying exercise intensities. It takes longer for your body to get fat out of storage and burned for fuel. When you're cruising at an easy pace, your body has time to tap into and burn your fat stores. As you crank up the intensity, your body needs more quick-burning fuel, so it turns to carbs. But your body never uses one or the other exclusively, and if you want to lose weight, your main goal should be burning calories, which is what high-intensity exercise does best.

If burning more fat still sounds better to you, consider this: If you ride for an hour at an easy to moderate pace, you'll burn about 450 calories, 270 of them from fat. Now, let's say you ride vigorously for that same hour. You'll burn 640 calories, about 250 of them from fat. In the end you've burned nearly 200 more calories and almost equal amounts of fat. Which one would you suspect is better for weight loss?

BUILDING STRUCTURE

The most important element of training is structure. By taking all the other essential elements of training and putting them into an actionable plan, you can make a smooth ascent toward your goals.

It sounds so obvious, but a huge number of riders (if not the vast majority) don't employ much, if any, structure at all. Instead, they go out and ride the same intensity—generally between 80% and 84% max heart rate, hard enough to feel like work but not hard enough to boost top-end fitness nor easy enough to allow suitable recovery—on every ride and then wonder why they aren't making measurable progress.

Even the slightest bit of structure works amazingly well. Commit yourself to riding one day *very* easy, one day *very* hard, and one day long. Mix it up (or cross train) on other days, and take one day completely off. Ramp up your intensity and training gradually and consistently, and you're guaranteed to make gains.

For even better results, you can craft a training plan in which every ride has a goal, whether it's to build endurance or improve top-end speed. The following are some common training elements that deliver specific results:

BASE MILES

Picture your fitness as if it were a house. The bigger the footprint or foundation, the bigger a house you can build. The footprint in cycling is your aerobic fitness. To build yours, you need lots of "moderate miles," long steady cruising rides in the 65 to 84% range (ideally averaging around 70% or 4 RPE). These rides boost your capillary development, improve your fat-burning ability, and generally build endurance. Base mile rides should be about two hours in length and should leave you pleasantly tired immediately afterward but not sore or wiped out for the whole day. If they do, you're going too hard.

INTERVALS

Coaches talk a lot about "specificity of training." That's jargonspeak for training your body to do what you want it to do. For instance, if your goal is to get faster, your body has to get comfortable working harder than it typically does. To do that, you need to systematically push it out of its comfort zone again and again. That in a nutshell is what *intervals,* sustained efforts, are all about.

Let's say you want to ride your usual 20-mile loop at 17 MPH, but you currently can't manage more than 15 MPH. By doing shorter intervals of 1 to 3 miles at 17 MPH (or even higher), broken up by periods of recovery, your body eventually adapts to that faster pace, so you can sustain it for your entire loop.

Like all training, intervals are designed to achieve a specific goal, such as improving top end speed, aerobic endurance, or hill climbing performance. The following are some of the most common types of interval. When doing these, don't forget the most important "interval" of all, the recovery interval. Lots of cyclists brag about the effort they put into their intervals, but they shortchange their recovery intervals. The rest periods between hard pushes should be ridiculously easy—a 2, *maybe* a 3, on the RPE scale. Little girls with baskets on their bikes should be able to keep up with you.

VO2 max

This is the glass ceiling you and your bike are trying to smash through. "VO2 max" is a fancy way of saying the maximum amount of oxygen your body can use when you're riding as hard as you can. That means how much oxygenated blood your heart can pump, how much blood your vessels can deliver, and how much oxygen your muscles can use. The only way to raise your max is by taking it to the max—that's a 10 on the RPE scale—in the form of very short all-out efforts lasting 20 seconds to 2 minutes.

Lactate threshold (LT)

If VO2 max is the glass ceiling, lactate threshold is the drop ceiling that, for most of us, hangs lower than we'd like. Very simplistically, this is the point at which you cross over from an aerobic effort to an anaerobic effort. For reasons I will explain, you can't stay above your lactate threshold for very long before your muscles beg for mercy and start shutting down. Athletes spend a lot of time and effort training to raise their lactate threshold, so they can ride longer and harder at a lower heart rate in a more aerobic state.

There are lots of ways to train LT, including hill repeats (going up and down a climb that lasts 10 to 20 minutes) or shorter, repeated, 3 to 5 minute efforts that undulate right above and right below your threshold. LT efforts are done on an 8 on the RPE scale.

Tempo

These efforts hover just slightly above your comfort zone but under your threshold. Like riding with someone just slightly faster than you, tempo intervals push you to breathe harder and feel like you're working, but not so hard that your legs are burning or you need to scale back to catch your breath. That means working at about a 6 on the RPE scale. Tempo intervals typically last 10 to 40 minutes in duration. Tempo efforts improve your body's ability to clear lactic acid, so they raise your lactate threshold.

Sprint

Good sprinting is about more than going fast. It's having the power and muscular endurance to give it your all at the end of a long, hard ride (when most big sprints take place). To boost sprinting power, you need to practice just that: At the end of a long ride, shift to a big gear and give 100% for 30 seconds. Then rest and do it again and again and again. These are done at 10 RPE.

PUTTING IT ALL TOGETHER

As you've seen, there are many ways up the training mountain. You can measure heart rate, you can track power, you can follow training zones based on perceived effort or breathing. The method you choose is ultimately up to you. For the purposes of this book, James Herrera and I have crafted training zones that should be easy for everyone from the greenest novice to the most seasoned cyclist to understand.

Below are the zones. In the following chapter, you'll find sample training programs for weight loss, century (100-mile) riding, and 40K time trial racing based on these ranges.

- **Easy (Zone 1, RPE 1 to 2):** Light to no effort.
- **Cruising (Zone 2, RPE 3 to 4):** Breathing deep, steady, and relaxed. Aerobic or cruising pace. You could spend the entire duration of your ride at this pace.
- **Steady (Zone 3, RPE 5 to 6):** Slightly shorter, quicker breathing than aerobic pace, still under control. A tempo pace you might use to climb a long hill.
- **Brisk (Zone 4, RPE 7 to 8):** Short, quick, rhythmic breathing. You're at LT. This is sometimes considered a climbing pace for shorter hills.
- **Max (Zone 5, RPE 9 to 10):** Max is just what it sounds like, the fastest, strongest pace you can sustain for the duration of the effort. Breathing will be heavy, short, and rapid. While many people are often intimidated by the sheer thought of doing a maximal effort, don't be too worried. Short, sprintlike efforts are tough, but they are a great and fun way to add some intensity to any workout while shaking things up a bit by breaking up the routine. A few five- to ten-second sprints at the end of a workout will always leave you feeling like you really put an exclamation point at the end of the day's training.

THE TRAINING ZONE MATRIX AT A GLANCE

The following chart pulls all the training zones together, so you'll know exactly what intensity you should be riding at whether you're tracking watts or breathing rate. I suggest you write in your own heart rate zone for each level, to help you personalize this training zone matrix.

NO PAIN, NO GAIN? MAYBE

You've heard this one a million times, and have likely heard that it's not true just as often. Though it's been largely misused and misunderstood, at its essence, it's true.

What's essential is that you can discern between "good pain" and "bad pain." Bad pain is "Ow! Something's really wrong." It's the feeling you get when you twist an ankle, strain your back, or pull a muscle. There's nothing productive about bad pain. So you should stop exercising immediately and tend to making it better.

Good pain is "Ooo! My legs are burning, I'm huffing and puffing, I don't think I can take this one second longer." That's productive pain. It hurts because it's hard, but it's the kind of pain that leaves you with a big goofy smile on your face the moment you stop (like at the top of an impossible climb). Without a little good pain, you won't make many gains.

REST AND REGENERATION

If you remember nothing else, remember this: You make your biggest gains in performance when you're *not* riding. Why? Because hard riding breaks your body down and rest rebuilds it better than it was before.

If all you do is push, push, push, however, you never give yourself the opportunity to fully improve. Instead, you create a state of chronic stress, where you're not only not getting stronger, you may actually backslide and start seeing your performance slip as you become chronically fatigued. It's called "overtraining," and you don't have to be a professional rider to have it happen to you. In fact, coaches who work with both pros and everyday Janes and Joes tell me it's more common in their recreational athletes than the elites. I never really believed that . . . until it happened to me.

TRAINING ZONE MATRIX							
Zone	Effort	Pace	RPE	% of Max Heart Rate	Your Heart Rate Target (fill in)	Breath-ing	% of Lactate Thresh-old
1	Recovery	Easy	1–2	60–64		Light and relaxed	30–40
2	Aerobic	Cruising	3–4	65–74		Deep and steady	50–70
3	Tempo	Steady	5–6	75–84		Slightly labored	75–85
4	Lactate Thresh-old	Brisk	7–8	85–94		Short and rhythmic	85–95
5	VO2 Max	Max	9–10	95–100		Rapid and heavy	100–130

AVOIDING STRESS OVERLOAD

Soon after my daughter was born, I was training for some early-season mountain bike races. I was following a carefully crafted training plan filled with plenty of rest days, but I found myself feeling increasingly tired. As I groused to a longtime racer pal about how I'd come to dread riding, she plainly told me what I should have seen: "You're overtrained." It was a stark reminder that there's more to rest than a day off your bike.

Training is a form of physical stress. Sure, it's fun and makes a great escape from work. But your body responds to a hard hilly ride the same way it does to a big meeting with the boss: Your heart rate rises, you sweat, and you pump out adrenaline. So, even if you're dutifully taking recovery days in your training, you can still end up burned out if you have too much uncontrolled stress in the rest of your life. That's why amateur athletes are at a special risk for overtraining; while sometimes stressful training is a bike pro's job, weekend warriors are layering that training on top of their regular work life.

I can tell when I start crossing the threshold into overtraining by my moods. I'm irritable, and instead of feeling jazzed about getting out to exercise, I'm exhausted just thinking about it. For me, it's more of a mental state of being, but it is also often a physical phenomenon. Some signs that you're overtrained (usually you'll have a few):

- Achy and tired muscles
- Fatigue
- Bad mood or depression
- Headaches
- Trouble sleeping
- High morning heart rate (your heart rate should be lowest in the morning)
- Susceptibility to colds and minor ailments
- Usual workouts feel more difficult than usual
- Lack of appetite

To avoid overtraining, you need to manage stress on and off the bike. To keep yourself fresh and fit (and therefore fast):

Keep it fun

Riding your bike is supposed to be fun. If you've signed up for an event and it's stressing you out, that's not fun. Remember, you won't finish last—and even if you do, you'll get more applause than the person who finishes fourth or fifth, or thirty-seventh for that matter. People cheer for and respect every single person on a competitive field for having the guts to be there in the first place.

Scale back every four weeks

Training should be progressive, so you want to keep adding intensity and distance. But you can't just build and build forever. Once a month, schedule an easy week, where you reduce the overall intensity and volume and give your mind and body a mini-break.

Take a deep breath

Once or twice a day, close your eyes and take a deep breath through your nose and deep into your diaphragm so your belly rises. Slowly exhale through your nose and repeat five to six times. Deep, belly breathing slows your heart rate and automatically puts you in a relaxed state.

Ride with your slower friends

Sometimes it's hard to ride as easy as you should to really recover fully. The sun is shining, the sky is blue, that little voice in your head says, "Woo-hoo! Let's go!" and, oops, you went too hard again. Go for a joyride with your kids or some slower friends and that won't happen.

START FRESH

The most important rest period is right before a big event. Anyone who has ever sat through final exams knows about cramming, studying around the clock trying to stuff as much information as humanly possible into your head. That technique may have earned you an A in Art History 101, but it's a recipe for failure for your first (or thirty-first) bike race or event.

No matter how much training you have or haven't done leading up to the final event, you need to *taper,* reduce your training load, before the big event. By cutting back on your riding time, you give your body a chance to fully restock its glycogen (muscle fuel) stores, repair any damaged muscle fibers or connective tissue, and pump up production of your aerobic enzymes. By giving your body a chance to make its final adjustments, you can come out stronger and faster on the day of your event.

In a review of fifty studies published in the *International Journal of Sports Medicine,* researchers found that tapering improves performance by 3%. That's about a minute faster for a 40K (25-mile) time trial race.

The more intense your event, the longer your taper should be, since you need to be as fresh as possible to give a 100% effort. Generally speaking, plan to taper for the week before your event, riding about 50% less and resting more. It's also important to reduce training *volume* but not *intensity.* You need to include hard intervals during your taper to maintain top end fitness, but only do half or a third your usual number. Just enough to keep your legs sharp but not make them tired.

JUST DO IT

Once you know how to measure your efforts, you're ready to start metering out those efforts in a meaningful way—training! On first read, all these new terms and techniques may feel overwhelming, but remember this: Training is nothing more complicated than riding hard and/or long sometimes and riding short and/or easy other times to improve your fitness. As with everything that requires effort, the first step is the hardest. That's why I'm going to make it super easy for you. In the next chapter, you'll find step-by-step instructions for building a training plan, including three complete plans for reaching common cycling goals. Once you get the hang of it—and start reaping the rewards of your hard work—you'll be hooked.

6

Build Your Training Plan

Got Goals? Here's How to Reach Them

There's a saying in cycling circles that summer races are won in December. That's just a clever way of saying that the training you do all year—not just in the weeks before your important events—adds up to measurable success when it comes time to put your fitness to the test.

A Year of Riding

Now that you know what's involved in training, let's put together some programs you can actually do. We'll start by taking a bird's-eye view of an entire year of training and then offer some specific cycling plans as well as off-season training routines that will help you reach your personal best.

Periodization: A Natural Progression

Periodization—the timing of your efforts to peak for a goal—is the backbone of any training program. I like to think of periodization as the natural progression of a cycling season. During the spring months, you're excited to ride, so you get out and do increasingly long rides, throwing in more hard efforts as you get more fit. During the summer, you're flying. You ride that wave of fitness into the fall, and as the days grow shorter, you ride a little less until winter, when you take a break from the bike, hit the gym, and get ready to start the cycle all over again. Even if you don't race, you can still use these principles to get faster throughout the year and from year to year.

As coaches use it, periodization is simply planning specific types of workouts at different times of the year so you can peak (be in top form) for a specific event. Instead of riding hard year-round desperately trying to maintain top fitness (an impossible feat), you divide the training year into different phases, so you can work on general fitness and strength (specific exercises explained later in the chapter), build a cycling fitness base, compete and peak, recover, and repeat the cycle again next year.

Though you sometimes have to tweak your phases forward or back (i.e., start serious bike training earlier or later in the year) depending on when your goal events are, in general, a year of periodization looks like this:

Preseason Building (January–March)

It's time to start ramping up for the new year. At the beginning of the year, you'll still be doing plenty of general strength and fitness building. Hit the free weights and do whatever cross training you enjoy. Get on your bike as weather permits, logging more bike time as the days get longer (and warmer, in the northern states). By mid-March, you should be riding about four days a week to build your base. (These sample schedules are for people who ride recreationally but aren't necessarily racing or trying to peak for a specific event. They also assume cycling is your main love and what you want to be doing in the summer. If you love running and swimming, feel free to tweak to allow for more cross training.)

JANUARY SAMPLE WEEK	
Monday	Strength and flexibility training
Tuesday	Trainer or outside ride
Wednesday	Strength and flexibility training
Thursday	Off or easy cross training
Friday	Strength and flexibility training
Saturday	Trainer or ride
Sunday	Cross training

FEBRUARY SAMPLE WEEK	
Monday	Strength and flexibility training
Tuesday	Off
Wednesday	Spinning class or trainer or ride
Thursday	Strength and flexibility training
Friday	Spinning class or trainer or ride
Saturday	Cross training
Sunday	Cross training

MARCH SAMPLE WEEK	
Monday	Strength and flexibility training
Tuesday	Spinning class or trainer or ride or cross training
Wednesday	Strength and flexibility training
Thursday	Off
Friday	Spinning class or trainer or ride or cross training
Saturday	Trainer or ride
Sunday	Trainer or ride

Cycling Season (April–September)

The goal for this season is to just get on your bike and ride. Time to really rack up the miles and prepare for the events of the season. Most of your hard efforts come during these months. Plan on devoting two days a week to doing higher-intensity efforts like hill climbs or intervals. Maintain your muscle strength and bone health with some light lifting once or twice a week.

APRIL SAMPLE WEEK	
Monday	Easy ride or light strength and flexibility training
Tuesday	Interval ride
Wednesday	Light strength and flexibility training
Thursday	Off
Friday	Hilly ride
Saturday	Long ride
Sunday	Long ride or cardio cross training

MAY SAMPLE WEEK	
Monday	Easy ride
Tuesday	Interval ride
Wednesday	Light strength and flexibility training
Thursday	Tempo ride
Friday	Light strength and flexibility training
Saturday	Long ride with hills
Sunday	Long ride or cardio cross training

JUNE THROUGH SEPTEMBER SAMPLE WEEKS*	
Monday	Light strength and flexibility training
Tuesday	Hilly ride
Wednesday	Tempo ride
Thursday	Off or light strength and flexibility training
Friday	Easy ride
Saturday	Charity ride
Sunday	Easy ride or cardio cross training

*As we get older, especially as women, strength training year-round becomes more important to maintain the strength (and bone density) we have. Some women can get away with going down to once a week during prime riding season. Others find they need to stick to twice weekly.

Active Recovery (October)

Fall is a beautiful time to enjoy the fruits of your labor. Forget about training for a few weeks and just ride as you like or get off the bike and go for a hike.

OCTOBER SAMPLE WEEK	
Monday	Off
Tuesday	Easy ride
Wednesday	Cross training
Thursday	Light strength and flexibility training
Friday	Hilly ride
Saturday	Hike
Sunday	Long ride

Rebuilding (November-December)

Cycling is an "imbalanced" sport, so while your legs get really, really strong, other parts of you—like your abs, back, and arms—can get pretty weak. Take the final months of the year to build some balanced fitness. Pilates, yoga, strength training, and a little indoor cycling is a recipe for a perfect off-season.

NOVEMBER SAMPLE WEEK	
Monday	Strength and flexibility training
Tuesday	Cross training
Wednesday	Strength and flexibility training
Thursday	Spinning class or trainer or ride
Friday	Strength and flexibility training
Saturday	Cross training or trainer or ride
Sunday	Cross training

DECEMBER SAMPLE WEEK	
Monday	Strength and flexibility training
Tuesday	Cross training or trainer or ride
Wednesday	Strength and flexibility training
Thursday	Off or easy cross training
Friday	Strength and flexibility training
Saturday	Trainer or ride
Sunday	Cross training

In-Season Training

It's time to start actually training! To help you get going, I tapped one of my most trusted colleagues, James Herrera, owner of Performance Driven Coaching in Colorado Springs, who has helped thousands of athletes of all ages and fitness levels reach their goals. Here you'll find three eight-week plans: weight loss, century, and 40K time trial. Each plan will be outlined in two ways: One version clearly outlines and explains each step in the schedule; the other is for quick reference once you're familiar with the program.

You'll be following the five training zones outlined on page 105 (they'll be labeled by their pace in the plans). Each calendar block in the plan tells you what to do that day. To read the quick reference chart, take the sample day below for example: On Tuesday, it says you should ride for an hour and fifteen minutes at Cruising pace. During that ride, you should include three Steady intervals that are fifteen minutes in length, allowing yourself to fully recover (so you feel ready for the next push) between efforts. It's that easy.

Tuesday
1:15
Cruising+ 3×15 min. Steady

After finishing your training plan and reaching your goal, you need to recover and rebuild. Think of it as reverse tapering. You should get out and ride (easy spinning helps speed recovery by increasing circulation through the muscles); just take it easy the first week back, keeping hard efforts to a minimum. The training volume the week after your event should resemble the week before your event. Figure about two to three days of recovery per hour you spent racing or riding hard. If you're new to the sport, you may find that you have some residual fatigue in the weeks that follow and you fizzle out faster than usual during hard efforts. Be patient and ride it out. Once you fully recover, you'll come back stronger than ever.

WEIGHT LOSS PLAN

Weight loss is a simple function of two things, calories in and calories out. Think of it as a scale that measures energy balance in your life. On one side, we've got food and drink. That's your calories coming in. On the other side, we've got your calories being burned, which is composed of a combination of activity level and your basal metabolic rate (BMR), the amount of energy (calories) you burn just living and breathing.

The ultimate goal for weight management is to balance our caloric intake with our output. If we're taking in more thàn we're burning, guess what? The excess gets stored as fat. On the flip side, if we're burning more than we're taking in, then voilà, we start to shed the pounds.

In the last chapter, you learned that you burn about 450 calories during an hour of easy to moderate intensity cycling, and in the neighborhood of 640 calories during higher intensity riding. Now remember our scale and energy balance. By adding to your activity level, you're increasing the number of calories burned, so the pounds should trickle off. It takes 3,500 burned calories to lose one pound of body weight, so all your excess weight won't fall off overnight, but you should see steady progress.

The other side of your energy balance is caloric intake. If you fuel your rides properly—that is, eat a light snack and/or drink an energy drink for your long rides—you should be able to have energy to ride yet still burn more than you're taking in. Be careful not to reward yourself too much with food. Studies show that people who successfully lose weight and keep it off do it by increasing their exercise while also trimming intake.

One way to keep track of this whole process is a simple bathroom scale. First thing in the morning, after you use the bathroom, step on the scale to see how it's going. Take your body weight once a week. If things are moving in the right direction, you'll know your strategy is on track. If the needle's moving in the wrong direction, you can make modifications quickly before ounces turn into pounds. Just remember that a woman's weight naturally fluctuates a few pounds. You're looking for trends.

Making Progress

Weight loss takes time. So does cycling. This plan assumes you can ride five days a week. If you can't, try to do at least four for the best results. It also assumes you've been doing some riding on your own. If you're brand new to the bike, take four to six weeks to put some miles in your legs before starting a structured program. A good rule of thumb is to increase your current ride volume by no greater than 10% weekly. Although, if your current riding volume is less than six total hours per week, it's perfectly safe to add 25% to your total weekly time.

A good training plan will include *progression*. This plan will increase in volume and intensity as you adapt to the training load. This means your total weekly ride volume increases from four to five to six hours over the course of three weeks. It also means that time you spend at a given intensity is gradually increased given the same workout volume: e.g., if your hour-long Wednesday ride included three Steady intervals of eight minutes with a brief five-minute recovery period between intervals, you will progressively increase the intensity of this hour-long workout to include two fifteen-minute Steady intervals, for a total of thirty minutes at that intensity.

Your sample plan is eight weeks long and offers a variety of ride intensities. Both total weekly volume and time spent during workouts at intensities above your Cruising pace are increased over a three-week period. On week four, you get a recovery week to give your body time to rest, regenerate, and adapt to the training load. This easier training week is not meant for running around and exhausting yourself with home improvement projects. Recovery means recovery! It is one of the most often neglected concepts in the training process and one of the primary reasons riders fail to see progress.

As you reach the end of your eight-week cycle, and you're wondering where to go from here, think about the concepts you've just learned. If you want to keep improving (and maybe speed weight loss), you'll need to keep progressing. If you have time, you can lengthen your rides. You can also increase intensity. Make your Steady intervals Brisk and toss in some short Max intervals. Or add hills. Remember to respect your recovery days and scale back every few weeks—trim your weekly volume by about a third and limit efforts to Easy and Cruising—to give your body time to completely regenerate. Continue progressing throughout the season, then take a break from the bike and enjoy some cross training when the weather turns. Next season, start it all up again.

The Weight Loss Plan at a Glance

This plan isn't designed for "racers," but that doesn't mean it's easy either. The most effective way to lose weight is to add intensity, so you will be working hard on some days. If you are new to the sport and find this plan too intense to start, simply lower the intensity on the intervals (e.g., doing Steady instead of Brisk).

WEEKS 1–4

W E E K	Mon-day	Tuesday	Wednes-day	Thursday	Friday	Saturday	Sunday
1	Rest day	1:00 Cruising + 20 min. Steady	1:00 Cruising	1:00 Cruising + 15 min. Brisk	0:30 Easy or full rest day	1:15 Cruising + 15 min. Steady and 10 min. Brisk	1:45 Cruising
2	Rest day	1:00 Cruising + 25 min. Steady	1:00 Cruising	1:00 Cruising + 20 min. Brisk	0:30 Easy or full rest day	1:30 Cruising + 20 min. Steady and 10 min. Brisk	1:45 Cruising
3	Rest day	1:00 Cruising + 30 min. Steady	1:00 Cruising	1:00 Cruising + 20 min. Brisk	0:30 Easy or full rest day	1:45 Cruising + 20 min. Steady and 15 min. Brisk	2:00 Cruising
4	Rest day	0:45 Cruising	0:30 Easy	0:45 Cruising	Rest day	1:15 Cruising	1:30 Cruising

WEEKS 5–8

WEEK	Monday	Tuesday	Wednesday	Thursday	Friday	Saturday	Sunday
5	Rest day	1:15 Cruising + 15 min. Steady and 10 min. Brisk	1:00 Cruising	1:15 Cruising + 10 min. Steady and 10 min. Brisk	0:45 Easy or full rest day	1:30 Cruising + 20 min. Steady and 15 min. Brisk	2:00 Cruising
6	Rest day	1:15 Cruising + 20 min. Steady and 10 min. Brisk	1:00 Cruising	1:15 Cruising + 15 min. Steady and 15 min. Brisk	0:45 Easy or full rest day	1:45 Cruising +25 min. Steady and 15 min. Brisk	2:15 Cruising
7	Rest day	1:15 Cruising + 25 min. Steady and 10 min. Brisk	1:00 Cruising	1:15 Cruising + 15 min. Steady and 20 min. Brisk	0:45 Easy or full rest day	2:00 Cruising + 30 min. Steady and 20 min. Brisk	2:15 Cruising
8	Rest day	1:00 Cruising	0:45 Easy	1:00 Cruising	Rest day	1:15 Cruising	1:30 Cruising

Weight Loss Plan Week by Week

One of the most common complaints I hear is that training plans are confusing to follow. I agree. So here is a detailed breakdown of what you should be doing on each day. If you have a heart rate monitor, you can photocopy these pages and write your personal heart rate numbers next to each entry. Please note that your heart rate does not respond instantaneously. Allow a little transition time between zones.

WEIGHT LOSS					WEEK 1, DAY 1
Goal for the day: Rest					
Plan for the day: Rest day—off to an easy start!					

WEIGHT LOSS					WEEK 1, DAY 2
Length: 1 hour					
Goal for the day: Hard					
Plan for the day: Cruising pace with 20 minutes at Steady pace					
Time	**Time elapse**	**Pace**	**Perceived Effort**	**% of Max**	**Your Heart Rate Target (fill in)**
0–20	20	Cruising	3–4	65–74%	
20–40	20	Steady	5–6	75-84%	
40–60	20	Cruising	3–4	65–74%	

WEIGHT LOSS					WEEK 1, DAY 3
Length: 1 hour					
Goal for the day: Easy					
Plan for the day: Cruising pace					
Time	**Time elapse**	**Pace**	**Perceived Effort**	**% of Max**	**Your Heart Rate Target (fill in)**
0–60	60	Cruising	3–4	65–74%	

WEIGHT LOSS					WEEK 1, DAY 4
Length: 1 hour					
Goal for the day: Hard					
Plan for the day: Cruising pace with 15 minutes at Brisk pace					
Time	Time elapse	Pace	Perceived Effort	% of Max	Your Heart Rate Target (fill in)
0–25	25	Cruising	3–4	65–74%	
25–40	15	Brisk	7–8	85–94%	
40–60	20	Cruising	3–4	65–74%	

WEIGHT LOSS					WEEK 1, DAY 5
Length: 30 minutes					
Goal for the day: Easy (or rest day)					
Plan for the day: Easy pace					
Time	Time elapse	Pace	Perceived Effort	% of Max	Your Heart Rate Target (fill in)
0–30	30	Easy	1–2	60–64%	

WEIGHT LOSS					WEEK 1, DAY 6
Length: 1 hour, 15 minutes					
Goal for the day: Hard					
Plan for the day: Cruising pace with 15 minutes at Steady pace and 10 minutes at Brisk pace					
Time	Time elapse	Pace	Perceived Effort	% of Max	Your Heart Rate Target (fill in)
0–15	15	Cruising	3–4	65–74%	
15–30	15	Steady	5–6	75–84%	
30–45	15	Cruising	3–4	65–74%	
45–55	10	Brisk	7–8	85–94%	
55–1:15	20	Cruising	3–4	65–74%	

WEIGHT LOSS					WEEK 1, DAY 7
Length: 1 hour, 45 minutes					
Goal for the day: Long					
Plan for the day: Cruising pace					
Time	Time elapse	Pace	Perceived Effort	% of Max	Your Heart Rate Target (fill in)
0–1:45	1:45	Cruising	3–4	65–74%	

WEIGHT LOSS	WEEK 2, DAY 1
Goal for the day: Rest	
Plan for the day: Rest day	

WEIGHT LOSS					WEEK 2, DAY 2
Length: 1 hour					
Goal for the day: Hard					
Plan for the day: Cruising pace with 25 minutes at Steady pace					
Time	Time elapse	Pace	Perceived Effort	% of Max	Your Heart Rate Target (fill in)
0–20	20	Cruising	3–4	65–74%	
20–45	25	Steady	5–6	75–84%	
45–60	15	Cruising	3–4	65–74%	

WEIGHT LOSS					WEEK 2, DAY 3
Length: 1 hour					
Goal for the day: Easy					
Plan for the day: Cruising pace					
Time	Time elapse	Pace	Perceived Effort	% of Max	Your Heart Rate Target (fill in)
0–60	60	Cruising	3–4	65–74%	

WEIGHT LOSS					WEEK 2, DAY 4
Length: 1 hour					
Goal for the day: Hard					
Plan for the day: Cruising pace with 20 minutes at Brisk pace					
Time	Time elapse	Pace	Perceived Effort	% of Max	Your Heart Rate Target (fill in)
0–20	20	Cruising	3–4	65–74%	
20–40	20	Brisk	7–8	85–94%	
40–60	20	Cruising	3–4	65–74%	

WEIGHT LOSS					WEEK 2, DAY 5
Length: 30 minutes (or rest day)					
Goal for the day: Easy					
Plan for the day: Easy pace					
Time	Time elapse	Pace	Perceived Effort	% of Max	Your Heart Rate Target (fill in)
0–30	30	Easy	1–2	60–64%	

WEIGHT LOSS					WEEK 2, DAY 6
Length: 1 hour, 30 minutes					
Goal for the day: Hard					
Plan for the day: Cruising pace with 20 minutes at Steady pace and 10 minutes at Brisk pace					
Time	Time elapse	Pace	Perceived Effort	% of Max	Your Heart Rate Target (fill in)
0–20	20	Cruising	3–4	65–74%	
20–40	20	Steady	5–6	75–84%	
40–60	20	Cruising	3–4	65–74%	
60–1:10	10	Brisk	7–8	85–94%	
1:10–1:30	20	Cruising	3–4	65–74%	

WEIGHT LOSS					WEEK 2, DAY 7
Length: 1 hour, 45 minutes					
Goal for the day: Long					
Plan for the day: Cruising pace					
Time	Time elapse	Pace	Perceived Effort	% of Max	Your Heart Rate Target (fill in)
0–1:45	1:45	Cruising	3–4	65–74%	

WEIGHT LOSS	WEEK 3, DAY 1
Goal for the day: Rest	
Plan for the day: Rest day	

WEIGHT LOSS					WEEK 3, DAY 2
Length: 1 hour					
Goal for the day: Hard					
Plan for the day: Cruising pace with 30 minutes at Steady pace					
Time	Time elapse	Pace	Perceived Effort	% of Max	Your Heart Rate Target (fill in)
0–15	15	Cruising	3–4	65–74%	
15–45	30	Steady	5–6	75–84%	
45–60	15	Cruising	3–4	65–74%	

WEIGHT LOSS					WEEK 3, DAY 3
Length: 1 hour					
Goal for the day: Easy					
Plan for the day: Cruising pace					
Time	Time elapse	Pace	Perceived Effort	% of Max	Your Heart Rate Target (fill in)
0–60	60	Cruising	3–4	65–74%	

WEIGHT LOSS					WEEK 3, DAY 4
Length: 1 hour					
Goal for the day: Hard					
Plan for the day: Cruising pace with 20 minutes at Brisk pace					
Time	Time elapse	Pace	Perceived Effort	% of Max	Your Heart Rate Target (fill in)
0–20	20	Cruising	3–4	65–74%	
20–40	20	Brisk	7–8	85–94%	
40–60	20	Cruising	3–4	65–74%	

WEIGHT LOSS					WEEK 3, DAY 5
Length: 30 minutes (or rest day)					
Goal for the day: Easy					
Plan for the day: Easy pace					
Time	Time elapse	Pace	Perceived Effort	% of Max	Your Heart Rate Target (fill in)
0–30	30	Easy	1–2	60–64%	

WEIGHT LOSS					WEEK 3, DAY 6
Length: 1 hour, 45 minutes					
Goal for the day: Hard					
Plan for the day: Cruising pace with 20 minutes at Steady pace and 15 minutes at Brisk pace					
Time	Time elapse	Pace	Perceived Effort	% of Max	Your Heart Rate Target (fill in)
0–20	20	Cruising	3–4	65–74%	
20–40	20	Steady	5–6	75–84%	
40–60	20	Cruising	3–4	65–74%	
60–1:15	15	Brisk	7–8	85–94%	
1:15–1:45	30	Cruising	3–4	65–74%	

WEIGHT LOSS					WEEK 3, DAY 7
Length: 2 hours					
Goal for the day: Long					
Plan for the day: Cruising pace					
Time	Time elapse	Pace	Perceived Effort	% of Max	Your Heart Rate Target (fill in)
0–2:00	2:00	Cruising	3–4	65–74%	

WEIGHT LOSS	WEEK 4, DAY 1
Goal for the day: Rest	
Plan for the day: Rest day	

WEIGHT LOSS					WEEK 4, DAY 2
Length: 45 minutes					
Goal for the day: Easy					
Plan for the day: Cruising pace					
Time	Time elapse	Pace	Perceived Effort	% of Max	Your Heart Rate Target (fill in)
0–45	45	Cruising	3–4	65–74%	

WEIGHT LOSS					WEEK 4, DAY 3
Length: 30 minutes					
Goal for the day: Easy					
Plan for the day: Easy pace					
Time	Time elapse	Pace	Perceived Effort	% of Max	Your Heart Rate Target (fill in)
0–30	30	Easy	1–2	60–64%	

WEIGHT LOSS					WEEK 4, DAY 4
Length: 45 minutes					
Goal for the day: Easy					
Plan for the day: Cruising pace					
Time	Time elapse	Pace	Perceived Effort	% of Max	Your Heart Rate Target (fill in)
0–45	45	Cruising	3–4	65–74%	

WEIGHT LOSS	WEEK 4, DAY 5
Goal for the day: Rest	
Plan for the day: Rest day	

WEIGHT LOSS					WEEK 4, DAY 6
Length: 1 hour, 15 minutes					
Goal for the day: Easy					
Plan for the day: Cruising pace					
Time	Time elapse	Pace	Perceived Effort	% of Max	Your Heart Rate Target (fill in)
0–1:15	1:15	Cruising	3–4	65–74%	

WEIGHT LOSS					WEEK 4, DAY 7
Length: 1 hour, 30 minutes					
Goal for the day: Long					
Plan for the day: Cruising pace					
Time	Time elapse	Pace	Perceived Effort	% of Max	Your Heart Rate Target (fill in)
0–1:30	1:30	Cruising	3–4	65–74%	

WEIGHT LOSS	WEEK 5, DAY 1
Goal for the day: Rest	
Plan for the day: Rest day	

WEIGHT LOSS					WEEK 5, DAY 2
Length: 1 hour, 15 minutes					
Goal for the day: Hard					
Plan for the day: Cruising pace with 15 minutes at Steady pace and 10 minutes at Brisk pace					
Time	Time elapse	Pace	Perceived Effort	% of Max	Your Heart Rate Target (fill in)
0–15	15	Cruising	3–4	65–74%	
15–30	15	Steady	5–6	75–84%	
30–45	15	Cruising	3–4	65–74%	
45–55	10	Brisk	7–8	85–94%	
55–1:15	20	Cruising	3–4	65–74%	

WEIGHT LOSS					WEEK 5, DAY 3
Length: 1 hour					
Goal for the day: Easy					
Plan for the day: Cruising pace					
Time	Time elapse	Pace	Perceived Effort	% of Max	Your Heart Rate Target (fill in)
0–60	60	Cruising	3–4	65–74%	

WEIGHT LOSS					WEEK 5, DAY 4
Length: 1 hour, 15 minutes					
Goal for the day: Hard					
Plan for the day: Cruising pace with 10 minutes at Steady pace and 10 minutes at Brisk pace					
Time	Time elapse	Pace	Perceived Effort	% of Max	Your Heart Rate Target (fill in)
0–20	20	Cruising	3–4	65–74%	
20–30	10	Steady	5–6	75–84%	
30–45	15	Cruising	3–4	65–74%	
45–55	10	Brisk	7–8	85–94%	
55–1:15	20	Cruising	3–4	65–74%	

WEIGHT LOSS					WEEK 5, DAY 5
Length: 45 minutes (or rest day)					
Goal for the day: Easy					
Plan for the day: Easy pace					
Time	Time elapse	Pace	Perceived Effort	% of Max	Your Heart Rate Target (fill in)
0–45	45	Easy	1–2	60–64%	

WEIGHT LOSS					WEEK 5, DAY 6
Length: 1 hour, 30 minutes					
Goal for the day: Hard					
Plan for the day: Cruising pace with 20 minutes at Steady pace and 15 minutes at Brisk pace					
Time	Time elapse	Pace	Perceived Effort	% of Max	Your Heart Rate Target (fill in)
0–20	20	Cruising	3–4	65–74%	
20–40	20	Steady	5–6	75–84%	
40–60	20	Cruising	3–4	65–74%	
60–1:15	15	Brisk	7–8	85–94%	
1:15–1:30	15	Cruising	3–4	65–74%	

WEIGHT LOSS					**WEEK 5, DAY 7**
Length: 2 hours					
Goal for the day: Long					
Plan for the day: Cruising pace					
Time	**Time elapse**	**Pace**	**Perceived Effort**	**% of Max**	**Your Heart Rate Target (fill in)**
0–2:00	2:00	Cruising	3–4	65–74%	

WEIGHT LOSS	**WEEK 6, DAY 1**
Goal for the day: Rest	
Plan for the day: Rest day	

WEIGHT LOSS					**WEEK 6, DAY 2**
Length: 1 hour, 15 minutes					
Goal for the day: Hard					
Plan for the day: Cruising pace with 20 minutes at Steady pace and 10 minutes at Brisk pace					
Time	**Time elapse**	**Pace**	**Perceived Effort**	**% of Max**	**Your Heart Rate Target (fill in)**
0–15	15	Cruising	3–4	65–74%	
15–35	20	Steady	5–6	75–84%	
35–50	15	Cruising	3–4	65–74%	
50–60	10	Brisk	7–8	85–94%	
60–1:15	15	Cruising	3–4	65–74%	

WEIGHT LOSS					WEEK 6, DAY 3
Length: 1 hour					
Goal for the day: Easy					
Plan for the day: Cruising pace					
Time	Time elapse	Pace	Perceived Effort	% of Max	Your Heart Rate Target (fill in)
0–60	60	Cruising	3–4	65–74%	

WEIGHT LOSS					WEEK 6, DAY 4
Length: 1 hour, 15 minutes					
Goal for the day: Hard					
Plan for the day: Cruising pace with 15 minutes at Steady pace and 15 minutes at Brisk pace					
Time	Time elapse	Pace	Perceived Effort	% of Max	Your Heart Rate Target (fill in)
0–15	15	Cruising	3–4	65–74%	
15–30	15	Steady	5–6	75–84%	
30–45	15	Cruising	3–4	65–74%	
45–60	15	Brisk	7–8	85–94%	
60–1:15	15	Cruising	3–4	65–74%	

WEIGHT LOSS					WEEK 6, DAY 5
Length: 45 minutes (or rest day)					
Goal for the day: Easy					
Plan for the day: Easy pace					
Time	Time elapse	Pace	Perceived Effort	% of Max	Your Heart Rate Target (fill in)
0–45	45	Easy	1–2	60–64%	

WEIGHT LOSS					WEEK 6, DAY 6
Length: 1 hour, 45 minutes					
Goal for the day: Hard					
Plan for the day: Cruising pace with 25 minutes at Steady pace and 15 minutes at Brisk pace					
Time	Time elapse	Pace	Perceived Effort	% of Max	Your Heart Rate Target (fill in)
0–20	20	Cruising	3–4	65–74%	
20–45	25	Steady	5–6	75–84%	
45–60	15	Cruising	3–4	65–74%	
60–1:15	15	Brisk	7–8	85–94%	
1:15–1:45	30	Cruising	3–4	65–74%	

WEIGHT LOSS					WEEK 6, DAY 7
Length: 2 hours, 15 minutes					
Goal for the day: Long					
Plan for the day: Cruising pace					
Time	Time elapse	Pace	Perceived Effort	% of Max	Your Heart Rate Target (fill in)
0–2:15	2:15	Cruising	3–4	65–74%	

WEIGHT LOSS	WEEK 7, DAY 1
Goal for the day: Rest	
Plan for the day: Rest day	

WEIGHT LOSS					WEEK 7, DAY 2
Length: 1 hour, 15 minutes					
Goal for the day: Hard					
Plan for the day: Cruising pace with 25 minutes at Steady pace and 10 minutes at Brisk pace					
Time	Time elapse	Pace	Perceived Effort	% of Max	Your Heart Rate Target (fill in)
0–15	15	Cruising	3–4	65–74%	
15–40	25	Steady	5–6	75–84%	
40–50	10	Cruising	3–4	65–74%	
50–60	10	Brisk	7–8	85–94%	
60–1:15	15	Cruising	3–4	65–74%	

WEIGHT LOSS					**WEEK 7, DAY 3**
Length: 1 hour					
Goal for the day: Easy					
Plan for the day: Cruising pace					
Time	**Time elapse**	**Pace**	**Perceived Effort**	**% of Max**	**Your Heart Rate Target (fill in)**
0–60	60	Cruising	3–4	65–74%	

WEIGHT LOSS					**WEEK 7, DAY 4**
Length: 1 hour, 15 minutes					
Goal for the day: Hard					
Plan for the day: Cruising pace with 15 minutes at Steady pace and 20 minutes at Brisk pace					
Time	**Time elapse**	**Pace**	**Perceived Effort**	**% of Max**	**Your Heart Rate Target (fill in)**
0–15	15	Cruising	3–4	65–74%	
15–30	15	Steady	5–6	75–84%	
30–45	15	Cruising	3–4	65–74%	
45–1:05	20	Brisk	7–8	85–94%	
1:05–1:15	10	Cruising	3–4	65–74%	

WEIGHT LOSS					WEEK 7, DAY 5
Length: 45 minutes (or rest day)					
Goal for the day: Easy					
Plan for the day: Easy pace					
Time	Time elapse	Pace	Perceived Effort	% of Max	Your Heart Rate Target (fill in)
0–45	45	Easy	1–2	60–64%	

WEIGHT LOSS					WEEK 7, DAY 6
Length: 2 hours					
Goal for the day: Hard					
Plan for the day: Cruising pace with 30 minutes at Steady pace and 20 minutes at Brisk pace					
Time	Time elapse	Pace	Perceived Effort	% of Max	Your Heart Rate Target (fill in)
0–15	15	Cruising	3–4	65–74%	
15–45	30	Steady	5–6	75–84%	
45–1:15	30	Cruising	3–4	65–74%	
1:15–1:35	20	Brisk	7–8	85–94%	
1:35–2:00	25	Cruising	3–4	65–74%	

WEIGHT LOSS					**WEEK 7, DAY 7**
Length: 2 hours, 15 minutes					
Goal for the day: Long					
Plan for the day: Cruising pace					
Time	**Time elapse**	**Pace**	**Perceived Effort**	**% of Max**	**Your Heart Rate Target (fill in)**
0–2:15	2:15	Cruising	3–4	65–74%	

WEIGHT LOSS	**WEEK 8, DAY 1**
Goal for the day: Rest	
Plan for the day: Rest day	

WEIGHT LOSS					**WEEK 8, DAY 2**
Length: 1 hour					
Goal for the day: Easy					
Plan for the day: Cruising pace					
Time	**Time elapse**	**Pace**	**Perceived Effort**	**% of Max**	**Your Heart Rate Target (fill in)**
0–60	60	Cruising	3–4	65–74%	

WEIGHT LOSS					WEEK 8, DAY 3
Length: 45 minutes					
Goal for the day: Easy					
Plan for the day: Easy pace					
Time	Time elapse	Pace	Perceived Effort	% of Max	Your Heart Rate Target (fill in)
0–45	45	Easy	1–2	60–64%	

WEIGHT LOSS					WEEK 8, DAY 4
Length: 1 hour					
Goal for the day: Easy					
Plan for the day: Cruising pace					
Time	Time elapse	Pace	Perceived Effort	% of Max	Your Heart Rate Target (fill in)
0–60	60	Cruising	3–4	65–74%	

WEIGHT LOSS	WEEK 8, DAY 5
Goal for the day: Rest	
Plan for the day: Rest day	

WEIGHT LOSS					WEEK 8, DAY 6
Length: 1 hour, 15 minutes					
Goal for the day: Easy					
Plan for the day: Cruising pace					
Time	Time elapse	Pace	Perceived Effort	% of Max	Your Heart Rate Target (fill in)
0–1:15	1:15	Cruising	3–4	65–74%	

WEIGHT LOSS					WEEK 8, DAY 7
Length: 1 hour, 30 minutes					
Goal for the day: Long					
Plan for the day: Cruising pace					
Time	Time elapse	Pace	Perceived Effort	% of Max	Your Heart Rate Target (fill in)
0–1:30	1:30	Cruising	3–4	65–74%	

  # CENTURY PLAN

A century event is a popular benchmark of cycling achievement. It seems to be a rite of passage to say, "Yes, I've made it into the club!" Whether it's your first or tenth century ride, a hundred miles on a bike is no small endeavor. Depending on your fitness and the severity of the terrain, you could be facing anywhere from five to ten hours in the saddle. Some mountain bike centuries push up into the twelve-hour mark. Now, that's a long day! Most popular road centuries in the

United States will keep an entry-level cyclist on his or her bike from seven to eight hours, intermediates from six to seven, and advanced riders from five to six. Advanced cyclists often try to break five hours, which means averaging 20 MPH for 100 miles—a huge endeavor. Whatever your goals or ability level may be, let's take it one step at a time.

IT ALL ADDS UP

A century plan includes progressively longer days in the saddle, especially on weekends. These rides are the perfect time to fine-tune your bike setup, gear selection, and food choices. A bike that feels fine for a twenty-mile jaunt might leave you with an achy back after five hours in the saddle. A good bike fit from a reputable shop or sports medicine clinic is well worth the investment. It's also time to work on the most important factors for century success: fueling and pacing.

Done properly, 100 miles on your bike is a rather enjoyable experience. Done improperly, that last 20 to 30 miles can be one of the longest, most painful stretches of road in your life. Another rite of passage in cycling: We're all going to "bonk" (run out of energy from poor fueling) at least once during an epic ride. While it's a certainty that it will happen to us all, by understanding the concepts of fueling and pacing, we can fend off this beast many, many times.

First and foremost, you *must* consume carbohydrates during the course of the ride. The faster you go, the more fuel you'll need, because you'll be burning more. Aim for 30 to 60 grams of carbohydrate (the lower end for light riders, the higher end for larger riders) an hour.

Several companies have developed an array of prepackaged fuel sources, like bars and carbohydrate gels, that are portable to carry, easy to digest, and come in a wide variety of shapes, sizes, and flavors. On average, an energy bar consists of 200 to 250 calories and is formulated to deliver about 20 grams of carbohydrate, 10 grams of protein, and 10 grams of fat. Carbohydrate gels run in the 100 to 125 calorie range and consist of 25 to 30 grams of a more easily digestible and simple carbohydrate source.

While the bars and gels can certainly do the trick, eating things that taste good are part of the reason we ride so long and hard. Consider tossing in Fig Newtons, trail mix, your favorite bite-size candy bar, cookies, peanut butter and jelly, honey, fresh fruit, pastries, bagels, pretzels, and potato chips. Easily digestible forms of carbohydrate that taste good are more likely to be consumed versus a snazzy, chemically engineered bar. And let's face it, 100 miles is hard work! You've earned that bag of M&M'S, Snickers bar, and handful of chocolate chip cookies. Regardless what food items you choose, take the time to experiment with new snacks during training to get an indication of how both your energy level and digestive system will respond to your choices.

Fluid consumption is just as important as, if not more important than, food intake. Even minor dehydration hurts performance. Aim to consume at least one 20-ounce water bottle per hour while using a combination of sports drink and water. Sports drinks such as Gatorade serve a dual purpose for the century cyclist: hydration and carbohydrate intake. Most are formulated with a balanced mixture of carbohydrate, protein, and electrolytes that will keep the body hydrated and in motion.

For both foods and fluids, eat and drink early and often! A century is a long time to be on the bike. Most century rides have planned rest stops where you can fill your bottles and grab some food. Take full advantage of these stops. What you eat and drink during hours two and three of your event will dictate how you perform in hours four, five, six, and beyond. It's a much easier task to keep the fire going by being attentive to your fuel intake than it is to try to recharge an extinguishing flame.

A sample day is outlined below. Please keep in mind that energy intake is extremely variable, and depending on your size and the speed you ride, you may need fewer or more calories. This is meant to be a starting point for an average 140-pound woman riding about 16 MPH. You may need to tweak according to your specific needs.

Event morning

Eat a good breakfast that fills you up without leaving you stuffed. Oatmeal is the perfect pre-century meal because it's easy to digest, yet it gives even, lasting energy. Add a banana and some juice (and coffee, if you drink java), and you're ready to roll.

Rest stop #1 (20 miles)

You shouldn't be too depleted yet. A sports drink and a few bites of energy bar will provide the 30 to 60 grams of easily digested carbohydrates that you need to top off your tank.

Rest stop #2 (45 miles)

By now your muscle glycogen stores are significantly depleted. A peanut butter and jelly sandwich with some juice, fig bars, and a few potato chips is a good lunch.

Rest stop #3 (65 miles)

When riders hit the wall it's often here in no man's land. You're not close enough to being done to get juiced up. You're too far in to be fresh. Treat yourself to a small brownie, half a Milky Way bar, or some other tasty treat to give you a lift.

Rest stop #4 (85 miles)

Your sweat loss can really catch up to you here. It's important to have a sports drink right about now.

The finish

Whoo-hoo! Celebrate with a high-carb, moderate-protein meal within thirty minutes of stopping to restock your glycogen stores while your muscles are at their hungriest.

PACE YOURSELF

Each of your longer weekend training rides is an opportunity to gauge what type of pace you might hold for the duration of your event. As a general rule of thumb, build your pace gradually over the course of the event so your performance moves upward in a step-wise fashion. Obviously, this is easier said than done. Many riders (especially first-timers) get swept up in the excitement of the day, roll out like thunder, and end up finishing a whole lot slower than they started. It helps to find similar-paced riders to roll with, which shouldn't be difficult when you consider you'll be sharing the road with hundreds if not thousands of other riders.

THE CENTURY PLAN AT A GLANCE

This is a generic plan for tackling a 100-mile day, but centuries are anything but cookie cutter. Some are flatter than cornfields in Kansas while others cross enormous mountain passes. It's important to train on terrain that closely matches what you'll be riding.

WEEKS 1–4

WEEK	Monday	Tuesday	Wednesday	Thursday	Friday	Saturday	Sunday
1	Rest day	1:15 Cruising + 3 × 15 min. Steady	1:00 Cruising	1:15 Cruising + 2 × 20 min. Steady/Brisk (15 min. Steady, 5 min. Brisk)	0:30 Easy or full rest day	2:00 Cruising + 20 min. Steady and 3 × 10 min. Brisk	3:00 Cruising on event-focused route (e.g., hilly or flat)
2	Rest day	1:30 Cruising + 2 × 25 min. Steady	1:00 Cruising	1:30 Cruising + 2 × 25 min. Steady/Brisk (18 min. Steady, 7 min. Brisk)	0:30 Easy or full rest day	2:30 Cruising + 30 min. Steady and 3 × 15 min. Brisk	3:15 Cruising on event-focused route (e.g., hilly or flat)
3	Rest day	1:30 Cruising + 4 × 15 min. Steady	1:00 Cruising	1:30 Cruising + 2 × 30 min. Steady/ Brisk (20 min. Steady, 10 min. Brisk)	0:45 Easy or full rest day	2:45 Cruising + 40 min. Steady and 4 × 15 min. Brisk.	3:30 Cruising on event-focused route (e.g., hilly or flat)
4	Rest day	1:00 Cruising	0:45 Easy	1:00 Cruising	Rest day	1:30 Cruising	2:00 Cruising on event-focused route (e.g., hilly or flat)

(WEEKS 5–8)							
W E E K	**Monday**	**Tuesday**	**Wednesday**	**Thursday**	**Friday**	**Saturday**	**Sunday**
5	Rest day	1:30 Cruising + 2 × 25 min. Steady	1:00 Cruising	1:30 Cruising + 2 × 25 min. Steady/Brisk (15 min. Steady, 10 min. Brisk)	0:45 Easy or full rest day	2:30 Cruising + 30 min. Steady and 3 × 10 min. Brisk	3:30 Cruising on event-focused route (e.g., hilly or flat)
6	Rest day	1:30 Cruising + 3 × 20 min. Steady	1:15 Cruising	1:30 Cruising + 2 × 30 min. Steady/Brisk (20 min. Steady, 10 min. Brisk)	0:45 Easy or full rest day	2:30 Cruising + 40 min. Steady and 3 × 15 min. Brisk	4:00 Cruising on event-focused route (e.g., hilly or flat)
7	Rest day	1:30 Cruising + 2 × 30 min. Steady	1:15 Cruising	1:30 Cruising + 2 × 30 min. Steady/Brisk (15 min. Steady, 15 min. Brisk)	0:45 Easy or full rest day	2:00 Cruising + 50 min. Steady and 4 × 10 min. Brisk	5:00 Cruising on event-focused route (e.g., hilly or flat)
8	Rest day	1:00 Cruising + 2 × 10 min. Steady	Rest day	1:00 Cruising + 2 × 5 min. Steady and 2 × 5 min. Brisk	Rest day	1:00 Cruising + 2 × 3 min. Steady and 2 × 3 min. Brisk	**Event!**

CENTURY PLAN WEEK BY WEEK

Here is a detailed breakdown of what you should be doing on each day. If you have a heart rate monitor, you can photocopy these pages and write your personal heart rate numbers next to each entry.

CENTURY					WEEK 1, DAY 1
Goal for the day: Rest					
Plan for the day: Rest day—off to an easy start!					

CENTURY					WEEK 1, DAY 2
Length: 1 hour, 15 minutes					
Goal for the day: Hard					
Plan for the day: Cruising pace with 3 separate 15-minute intervals at Steady pace					

Time	Time elapse	Pace	Perceived Effort	% of Max	Your Heart Rate Target (fill in)
0–10	10	Cruising	3–4	65–74%	
10–25	15	Steady	5–6	75–84%	
25–30	5	Cruising	3–4	65–74%	
30–45	15	Steady	5–6	75–84%	
45–50	5	Cruising	3–4	65–74%	
50–1:05	15	Steady	5–6	75–84%	
1:05–1:15	10	Cruising	3–4	65–74%	

CENTURY					WEEK 1, DAY 3
Length: 1 hour					
Goal for the day: Easy					
Plan for the day: Cruising pace					
Time	Time elapse	Pace	Perceived Effort	% of Max	Your Heart Rate Target (fill in)
0–60	60	Cruising	3–4	65–74%	

CENTURY					WEEK 1, DAY 4
Length: 1 hour, 15 minutes					
Goal for the day: Hard					
Plan for the day: Cruising pace with 2 separate 20-minute intervals at Steady/ Brisk pace (15 minutes at Steady and 5 minutes at Brisk for each interval)					
Time	Time elapse	Pace	Perceived Effort	% of Max	Your Heart Rate Target (fill in)
0–15	15	Cruising	3–4	65–74%	
15–30	15	Steady	5–6	75–84%	
30–35	5	Brisk	7–8	85–94%	
35–45	10	Cruising	3–4	65–74%	
45–60	15	Steady	5–6	75–84%	
60–1:05	5	Brisk	7–8	85–94%	
1:05–1:15	10	Cruising	3–4	65–74%	

CENTURY					WEEK 1, DAY 5
Length: 30 minutes (or rest day)					
Goal for the day: Easy					
Plan for the day: Easy pace					
Time	**Time elapse**	**Pace**	**Perceived Effort**	**% of Max**	**Your Heart Rate Target (fill in)**
0–30	30	Easy	1–2	60–64%	

CENTURY					WEEK 1, DAY 6
Length: 2 hours					
Goal for the day: Hard					
Plan for the day: Cruising pace with 20 minutes at Steady pace and 3 separate 10-minute intervals at Brisk pace					
Time	**Time elapse**	**Pace**	**Perceived Effort**	**% of Max**	**Your Heart Rate Target (fill in)**
0–15	15	Cruising	3–4	65–74%	
15–35	20	Steady	5–6	75–84%	
35–45	10	Cruising	3–4	65–74%	
45–55	10	Brisk	7–8	85–94%	
55–1:10	15	Cruising	3–4	65–74%	
1:10–1:20	10	Brisk	7–8	85–94%	
1:20–1:30	10	Cruising	3–4	65–74%	
1:30–1:40	10	Brisk	7–8	85–94%	
1:40–2:00	20	Cruising	3–4	65–74%	

CENTURY					WEEK 1, DAY 7
Length: 3 hours					
Goal for the day: Long					
Plan for the day: Cruising pace					
Tip: Ride a route that is similar to your century route (e.g., hilly, rolling, flat)					
Time	**Time elapse**	**Pace**	**Perceived Effort**	**% of Max**	**Your Heart Rate Target (fill in)**
0–3:00	3:00	Cruising	3–4	65–74%	

CENTURY	WEEK 2, DAY 1
Goal for the day: Rest	
Plan for the day: Rest day	

CENTURY					WEEK 2, DAY 2
Length: 1 hour, 30 minutes					
Goal for the day: Hard					
Plan for the day: Cruising pace with 2 separate 25-minute intervals at Steady pace					
Time	**Time elapse**	**Pace**	**Perceived Effort**	**% of Max**	**Your Heart Rate Target (fill in)**
0–15	15	Cruising	3–4	65–74%	
15–40	25	Steady	5–6	75–84%	
40–50	10	Cruising	3–4	65–74%	
50–1:15	25	Steady	5–6	75–84%	
1:15–1:30	15	Cruising	3–4	65–74%	

CENTURY					WEEK 2, DAY 3

Length: 1 hour

Goal for the day: Easy

Plan for the day: Cruising pace

Time	Time elapse	Pace	Perceived Effort	% of Max	Your Heart Rate Target (fill in)
0–60	60	Cruising	3–4	65–74%	

CENTURY					WEEK 2, DAY 4

Length: 1 hour, 30 minutes

Goal for the day: Hard

Plan for the day: Cruising pace with 2 separate 25-minute intervals at Steady/ Brisk pace (18 minutes at Steady and 7 minutes at Brisk for each interval)

Time	Time elapse	Pace	Perceived Effort	% of Max	Your Heart Rate Target (fill in)
0–15	15	Cruising	3–4	65–74%	
15–33	18	Steady	5–6	75–84%	
33–40	7	Brisk	7–8	85–94%	
40–50	10	Cruising	3–4	65–74%	
50–1:08	18	Steady	5–6	75–84%	
1:08–1:15	7	Brisk	7–8	85–94%	
1:15–1:30	15	Cruising	3–4	65–74%	

CENTURY					WEEK 2, DAY 5

Length: 30 minutes (or rest day)

Goal for the day: Easy

Plan for the day: Easy pace

Time	Time elapse	Pace	Perceived Effort	% of Max	Your Heart Rate Target (fill in)
0–30	30	Easy	1–2	60–64%	

CENTURY					WEEK 2, DAY 6
Length: 2 hours, 30 minutes					
Goal for the day: Hard					
Plan for the day: Cruising pace with 30 minutes at Steady pace and 3 separate 15-minute intervals at Brisk pace					
Time	Time elapse	Pace	Perceived Effort	% of Max	Your Heart Rate Target (fill in)
0–15	15	Cruising	3–4	65–74%	
15–45	30	Steady	5–6	75–84%	
45–60	15	Cruising	3–4	65–74%	
60–1:15	15	Brisk	7–8	85–94%	
1:15–1:30	15	Cruising	3–4	65–74%	
1:30–1:45	15	Brisk	7–8	85–94%	
1:45–2:00	15	Cruising	3–4	65–74%	
2:00–2:15	15	Brisk	7–8	85–94%	
2:15–2:30	15	Cruising	3–4	65–74%	

CENTURY					WEEK 2, DAY 7
Length: 3 hours, 15 minutes					
Goal for the day: Long					
Plan for the day: Cruising pace **Tip: Ride a route that is similar to your Century route (e.g., hilly, rolling, flat)**					
Time	Time elapse	Pace	Perceived Effort	% of Max	Your Heart Rate Target (fill in)
0–3:15	3:15	Cruising	3–4	65–74%	

CENTURY					WEEK 3, DAY 1
Goal for the day: Rest					
Plan for the day: Rest day					

CENTURY					WEEK 3, DAY 2
Length: 1 hour, 30 minutes					
Goal for the day: Hard					
Plan for the day: Cruising pace with 4 separate 15-minute intervals at Steady pace					
Time	**Time elapse**	**Pace**	**Perceived Effort**	**% of Max**	**Your Heart Rate Target (fill in)**
0–10	10	Cruising	3–4	65–74%	
10–25	15	Steady	5–6	75–84%	
25–30	5	Cruising	3–4	65–74%	
30–45	15	Steady	5–6	75–84%	
45–50	5	Cruising	3–4	65–74%	
50–1:05	15	Steady	5–6	75–84%	
1:05–1:10	5	Cruising	3–4	65–74%	
1:10–1:25	15	Steady	5–6	75–84%	
1:25–1:30	5	Cruising	3–4	65–74%	

CENTURY					WEEK 3, DAY 3
Length: 1 hour					
Goal for the day: Easy					
Plan for the day: Cruising pace					
Time	**Time elapse**	**Pace**	**Perceived Effort**	**% of Max**	**Your Heart Rate Target (fill in)**
0–60	60	Cruising	3–4	65–74%	

CENTURY					WEEK 3, DAY 4
Length: 1 hour, 30 minutes					
Goal for the day: Hard					
Plan for the day: Cruising pace with 2 separate 30-minute intervals at Steady/ Brisk pace (20 minutes at Steady and 10 minutes at Brisk for each interval)					
Time	Time elapse	Pace	Perceived Effort	% of Max	Your Heart Rate Target (fill in)
0–10	10	Cruising	3–4	65–74%	
10–30	20	Steady	5–6	75–84%	
30–40	10	Brisk	7–8	85–94%	
40–50	10	Cruising	3–4	65–74%	
50–1:10	20	Steady	5–6	75–84%	
1:10–1:20	10	Brisk	7–8	85–94%	
1:20–1:30	10	Cruising	3–4	65–74%	

CENTURY					WEEK 3, DAY 5
Length: 45 minutes (or rest day)					
Goal for the day: Easy					
Plan for the day: Easy pace					
Time	Time elapse	Pace	Perceived Effort	% of Max	Your Heart Rate Target (fill in)
0–45	45	Easy	1–2	60–64%	

CENTURY					WEEK 3, DAY 6

Length: 2 hours, 45 minutes

Goal for the day: Hard

Plan for the day: Cruising pace with 40 minutes at Steady pace and 4 separate 15-minute intervals at Brisk pace

Time	Time elapse	Pace	Perceived Effort	% of Max	Your Heart Rate Target (fill in)
0–15	15	Cruising	3–4	65–74%	
15–55	40	Steady	5–6	75–84%	
55–1:05	10	Cruising	3–4	65–74%	
1:05–1:20	15	Brisk	7–8	85–94%	
1:20–1:30	10	Cruising	3–4	65–74%	
1:30–1:45	15	Brisk	7–8	85–94%	
1:45–1:55	10	Cruising	3–4	65–74%	
1:55–2:10	15	Brisk	7–8	85–94%	
2:10–2:20	10	Cruising	3–4	65–74%	
2:20–2:35	15	Brisk	7–8	85–94%	
2:35–2:45	10	Cruising	3–4	65–74%	

CENTURY					WEEK 3, DAY 7

Length: 3 hours, 30 minutes

Goal for the day: Long

Plan for the day: Cruising pace
Tip: Ride a route that is similar to your century route (e.g., hilly, rolling, flat)

Time	Time elapse	Pace	Perceived Effort	% of Max	Your Heart Rate Target (fill in)
0–3:30	3:30	Cruising	3–4	65–74%	

CENTURY					WEEK 4, DAY 1
Goal for the day: Rest					
Plan for the day: Rest day					

CENTURY					WEEK 4, DAY 2
Length: 1 hour					
Goal for the day: Easy					
Plan for the day: Cruising pace					
Time	Time elapse	Pace	Perceived Effort	% of Max	Your Heart Rate Target (fill in)
0–1:00	1:00	Cruising	3–4	65–74%	

CENTURY					WEEK 4, DAY 3
Length: 45 minutes					
Goal for the day: Easy					
Plan for the day: Easy pace					
Time	Time elapse	Pace	Perceived Effort	% of Max	Your Heart Rate Target (fill in)
0–45	45	Easy	1–2	60–64%	

CENTURY					WEEK 4, DAY 4
Length: 1 hour					
Goal for the day: Easy					
Plan for the day: Cruising pace					
Time	Time elapse	Pace	Perceived Effort	% of Max	Your Heart Rate Target (fill in)
0–1:00	1:00	Cruising	3–4	65–74%	

CENTURY	WEEK 4, DAY 5
Goal for the day: Rest	
Plan for the day: Rest day	

CENTURY					WEEK 4, DAY 6
Length: 1 hour, 30 minutes					
Goal for the day: Easy					
Plan for the day: Cruising pace					
Time	Time elapse	Pace	Perceived Effort	% of Max	Your Heart Rate Target (fill in)
0–1:30	1:30	Cruising	3–4	65–74%	

CENTURY					WEEK 4, DAY 7
Length: 2 hours					
Goal for the day: Long					
Plan for the day: Cruising pace					
Tip: Ride a route that is similar to your century route (e.g., hilly, rolling, flat)					
Time	Time elapse	Pace	Perceived Effort	% of Max	Your Heart Rate Target (fill in)
0–2:00	2:00	Cruising	3–4	65–74%	

CENTURY	WEEK 5, DAY 1
Goal for the day: Rest	
Plan for the day: Rest day	

CENTURY					WEEK 5, DAY 2
Length: 1 hour, 30 minutes					
Goal for the day: Hard					
Plan for the day: Cruising pace with 2 separate 25-minute intervals at Steady pace					
Time	Time elapse	Pace	Perceived Effort	% of Max	Your Heart Rate Target (fill in)
0–15	15	Cruising	3–4	65–74%	
15–40	25	Steady	5–6	75–84%	
40–50	10	Cruising	3–4	65–74%	
50–1:15	25	Steady	5–6	75–84%	
1:15–1:30	15	Cruising	3–4	65–74%	

CENTURY					WEEK 5, DAY 3
Length: 1 hour					
Goal for the day: Easy					
Plan for the day: Cruising pace					
Time	Time elapse	Pace	Perceived Effort	% of Max	Your Heart Rate Target (fill in)
0–1:00	1:00	Cruising	3–4	65–74%	

CENTURY					WEEK 5, DAY 4
Length: 1 hour, 30 minutes					
Goal for the day: Hard					
Plan for the day: Cruising pace with 2 separate 25-minute intervals at Steady/ Brisk pace (15 minutes at Steady and 10 minutes at Brisk for each interval)					
Time	**Time elapse**	**Pace**	**Perceived Effort**	**% of Max**	**Your Heart Rate Target (fill in)**
0–15	15	Cruising	3–4	65–74%	
15–30	15	Steady	5–6	75–84%	
30–40	10	Brisk	7–8	85–94%	
40–50	10	Cruising	3–4	65–74%	
50–1:05	15	Steady	5–6	75–84%	
1:05–1:15	10	Brisk	7–8	85–94%	
1:15–1:30	15	Cruising	3–4	65–74%	

CENTURY					WEEK 5, DAY 5
Length: 45 minutes (or rest day)					
Goal for the day: Easy					
Plan for the day: Easy pace					
Time	**Time elapse**	**Pace**	**Perceived Effort**	**% of Max**	**Your Heart Rate Target (fill in)**
0–45	45	Easy	1–2	60–64%	

CENTURY					WEEK 5, DAY 6
Length: 2 hours, 30 minutes					
Goal for the day: Hard					
Plan for the day: Cruising pace with 30 minutes at Steady pace and 3 separate 10-minute intervals at Brisk pace					
Time	Time elapse	Pace	Perceived Effort	% of Max	Your Heart Rate Target (fill in)
0–15	15	Cruising	3–4	65–74%	
15–45	30	Steady	5–6	75–84%	
45–60	15	Cruising	3–4	65–74%	
60–1:10	10	Brisk	7–8	85–94%	
1:10–1:25	15	Cruising	3–4	65–74%	
1:25–1:35	10	Brisk	7–8	85–94%	
1:35–1:50	15	Cruising	3–4	65–74%	
1:50–2:00	10	Brisk	7–8	85–94%	
2:00–2:30	30	Cruising	3–4	65–74%	

CENTURY					WEEK 5, DAY 7
Length: 3 hours, 30 minutes					
Goal for the day: Long					
Plan for the day: Cruising pace					
Tip: Ride a route that is similar to your century route (e.g., hilly, rolling, flat)					
Time	Time elapse	Pace	Perceived Effort	% of Max	Your Heart Rate Target (fill in)
0–3:30	3:30	Cruising	3–4	65–74%	

CENTURY					WEEK 6, DAY 1
Goal for the day: Rest					
Plan for the day: Rest day					

CENTURY					WEEK 6, DAY 2
Length: 1 hour, 30 minutes					
Goal for the day: Hard					
Plan for the day: Cruising pace with 3 separate 20-minute intervals at Steady pace					
Time	**Time elapse**	**Pace**	**Perceived Effort**	**% of Max**	**Your Heart Rate Target (fill in)**
0–10	10	Cruising	3–4	65–74%	
10–30	20	Steady	5–6	75–84%	
30–35	5	Cruising	3–4	65–74%	
35–55	20	Steady	5–6	75–84%	
55–60	5	Cruising	3–4	65–74%	
60–1:20	20	Steady	5–6	74–84%	
1:20–1:30	10	Cruising	3–4	65–74%	

CENTURY					WEEK 6, DAY 3
Length: 1 hour, 15 minutes					
Goal for the day: Easy					
Plan for the day: Cruising pace					
Time	**Time elapse**	**Pace**	**Perceived Effort**	**% of Max**	**Your Heart Rate Target (fill in)**
0–1:15	1:15	Cruising	3–4	65–74%	

CENTURY					WEEK 6, DAY 4
Length: 1 hour, 30 minutes					
Goal for the day: Hard					
Plan for the day: Cruising pace with 2 separate 30-minute intervals at Steady/ Brisk pace (20 minutes at Steady and 10 minutes at Brisk for each interval)					
Time	Time elapse	Pace	Perceived Effort	% of Max	Your Heart Rate Target (fill in)
0–10	10	Cruising	3–4	65–74%	
10–30	20	Steady	5–6	75–84%	
30–40	10	Brisk	7–8	85–94%	
40–50	10	Cruising	3–4	65–74%	
50–1:10	20	Steady	5–6	75–84%	
1:10–1:20	10	Brisk	7–8	85–94%	
1:20–1:30	10	Cruising	3–4	65–74%	

CENTURY					WEEK 6, DAY 5
Length: 45 minutes (or rest day)					
Goal for the day: Easy					
Plan for the day: Easy pace					
Time	Time elapse	Pace	Perceived Effort	% of Max	Your Heart Rate Target (fill in)
0–45	45	Easy	1–2	60–64%	

CENTURY					WEEK 6, DAY 6
Length: 2 hours, 30 minutes					
Goal for the day: Hard					
Plan for the day: Cruising pace with 40 minutes at Steady pace and 3 separate 15-minute intervals at Brisk pace					
Time	**Time elapse**	**Pace**	**Perceived Effort**	**% of Max**	**Your Heart Rate Target (fill in)**
0–15	15	Cruising	3–4	65–74%	
15–55	40	Steady	5–6	75–84%	
55–1:10	15	Cruising	3–4	65–74%	
1:10–1:25	15	Brisk	7–8	85–94%	
1:25–1:35	10	Cruising	3–4	65–74%	
1:35–1:50	15	Brisk	7–8	85–94%	
1:50–2:00	10	Cruising	3–4	65–74%	
2:00–2:15	15	Brisk	7–8	85–94%	
2:15–2:30	15	Cruising	3–4	65–74%	

CENTURY					WEEK 6, DAY 7
Length: 4 hours					
Goal for the day: Long					
Plan for the day: Cruising pace					
Tip: Ride a route that is similar to your century route (e.g., hilly, rolling, flat)					
Time	**Time elapse**	**Pace**	**Perceived Effort**	**% of Max**	**Your Heart Rate Target (fill in)**
0–4:00	4:00	Cruising	3–4	65–74%	

CENTURY					WEEK 7, DAY 1
Goal for the day: Rest					
Plan for the day: Rest day					

CENTURY					WEEK 7, DAY 2
Length: 1 hour, 30 minutes					
Goal for the day: Hard					
Plan for the day: Cruising pace with 2 separate 30-minute intervals at Steady pace					

Time	Time elapse	Pace	Perceived Effort	% of Max	Your Heart Rate Target (fill in)
0–10	10	Cruising	3–4	65–74%	
10–40	30	Steady	5–6	75–84%	
40–50	10	Cruising	3–4	65–74%	
50–1:20	30	Steady	5–6	75–84%	
1:20–1:30	10	Cruising	3–4	65–74%	

CENTURY					WEEK 7, DAY 3
Length: 1 hour, 15 minutes					
Goal for the day: Easy					
Plan for the day: Cruising pace					

Time	Time elapse	Pace	Perceived Effort	% of Max	Your Heart Rate Target (fill in)
0–1:15	1:15	Cruising	3–4	65–74%	

CENTURY					WEEK 7, DAY 4
Length: 1 hour, 30 minutes					
Goal for the day: Hard					
Plan for the day: Cruising pace with 2 separate 30-minute intervals at Steady/ Brisk pace (15 minutes at Steady and 15 minutes at Brisk for each interval)					
Time	**Time elapse**	**Pace**	**Perceived Effort**	**% of Max**	**Your Heart Rate Target (fill in)**
0–10	10	Cruising	3–4	65–74%	
10–25	15	Steady	5–6	75–84%	
25–40	15	Brisk	7–8	85–94%	
40–50	10	Cruising	3–4	65–74%	
50–1:05	15	Steady	5–6	75–84%	
1:05–1:20	15	Brisk	7–8	85–94%	
1:20–1:30	10	Cruising	3–4	65–74%	

CENTURY					WEEK 7, DAY 5
Length: 45 minutes (or rest day)					
Goal for the day: Easy					
Plan for the day: Easy pace					
Time	**Time elapse**	**Pace**	**Perceived Effort**	**% of Max**	**Your Heart Rate Target (fill in)**
0–45	45	Easy	1–2	60–64%	

CENTURY					WEEK 7, DAY 6
Length: 2 hours					
Goal for the day: Hard					
Plan for the day: Cruising pace with 50 minutes at Steady pace and 4 separate 10-minute intervals at Brisk pace					
Time	Time elapse	Pace	Perceived Effort	% of Max	Your Heart Rate Target (fill in)
0–5	5	Cruising	3–4	65–74%	
5–55	50	Steady	5–6	75–84%	
55–60	5	Cruising	3–4	65–74%	
60–1:10	10	Brisk	7–8	85–94%	
1:10–1:15	5	Cruising	3–4	65–74%	
1:15–1:25	10	Brisk	7–8	85–94%	
1:25–1:30	5	Cruising	3–4	65–74%	
1:30–1:40	10	Brisk	7–8	85–94%	
1:40–1:45	5	Cruising	3–4	65–74%	
1:45–1:55	10	Brisk	7–8	85–94%	
1:55–2:00	5	Cruising	3–4	65–74%	

CENTURY					WEEK 7, DAY 7
Length: 5 hours					
Goal for the day: Long					
Plan for the day: Cruising pace **Tip: Ride a route that is similar to your century route (e.g., hilly, rolling, flat)**					
Time	Time elapse	Pace	Perceived Effort	% of Max	Your Heart Rate Target (fill in)
0–5:00	5:00	Cruising	3–4	65–74%	

CENTURY	WEEK 8, DAY 1
Goal for the day: Rest	
Plan for the day: Rest day	

CENTURY — **WEEK 8, DAY 2**

Length: 1 hour

Goal for the day: Hard

Plan for the day: Cruising pace with 2 separate 10-minute intervals at Steady pace

Time	Time elapse	Pace	Perceived Effort	% of Max	Your Heart Rate Target (fill in)
0–15	15	Cruising	3–4	65–74%	
15–25	10	Steady	5–6	75–84%	
25–35	10	Cruising	3–4	65–74%	
35–45	10	Steady	5–6	75–84%	
45–1:00	15	Cruising	3–4	65–74%	

CENTURY	WEEK 8, DAY 3
Goal for the day: Rest	
Plan for the day: Rest day	

CENTURY					WEEK 8, DAY 4
Length: 1 hour					
Goal for the day: Hard					
Plan for the day: Cruising pace with 2 separate 5-minute intervals at Steady pace and 2 separate 5-minute intervals at Brisk pace					
Time	Time elapse	Pace	Perceived Effort	% of Max	Your Heart Rate Target (fill in)
0–10	10	Cruising	3–4	65–74%	
10–15	5	Steady	5–6	75–84%	
15–20	5	Cruising	3–4	65–74%	
20–25	5	Brisk	7–8	85–94%	
25–30	5	Cruising	3–4	65–74%	
30–35	5	Steady	5–6	75–84%	
35–40	5	Cruising	3–4	65–74%	
40–45	5	Brisk	7–8	85–94%	
45–60	15	Cruising	3–4	65–74%	

CENTURY	WEEK 8, DAY 5
Goal for the day: Rest	
Plan for the day: Rest day	

CENTURY					WEEK 8, DAY 6
Length: 1 hour					
Goal for the day: Hard					
Plan for the day: Cruising pace with 2 separate 3-minute intervals at Steady pace and 2 separate 3-minute intervals at Brisk pace					
Time	Time elapse	Pace	Perceived Effort	% of Max	Your Heart Rate Target (fill in)
0–15	15	Cruising	3–4	65–74%	
15–18	3	Steady	5–6	75–84%	
18–25	7	Cruising	3–4	65–74%	
25–28	3	Brisk	7–8	85–94%	
28–35	7	Cruising	3–4	65–74%	
35–38	3	Steady	5–6	75–84%	
38–45	7	Cruising	3–4	65–74%	
45–48	3	Brisk	7–8	85–94%	
48–60	12	Cruising	3–4	65–74%	

CENTURY EVENT!	WEEK 8, DAY 7

 # 40K TIME TRIAL (TT)

A time trial is considered the "race of truth" as a cycling discipline. It is simply a rider racing the clock over a predetermined distance with the sole goal of posting the fastest time possible. The 40K distance (24.69 miles) is an incredibly popular and widely used format in national-level racing. Riders depart the start area in thirty-second to one-minute intervals, and all cover the exact same course.

TRAINING AND PACING

As with all event-specific training, it's critical to mimic the terrain you'll be racing on during your training. Simply put, if your time trial will be on rolling or uphill terrain, you don't want to do all your training on the flats. You want to gain power and leg speed on the bike that will transfer to your event.

It's also essential to train on your TT bike as much as possible. Use easier, noninterval training rides to begin working with your position on the bike, making adjustments in minor increments. A good bike fit can be the difference between comfortable blistering speed and a screaming back, so get a professional bike fit if possible. You'll need to get comfortable spending time in your tuck, eventually progressing toward doing harder TT-specific efforts on the bike. There's a number of progressive workouts imbedded in your 40K training plan to accomplish this task.

Finding your 40K pace during brisk training intervals is also an incredibly important goal. Successful time trialing is all about getting comfortable with the pain of your threshold pace. The quicker you can make peace with this pace or get comfortable with a slight bit of discomfort, the more successful your efforts will be. The majority of the time you'll be racing your 40K, you'll be in the throes of a brisk pace, hovering right at or slightly above your lactate threshold (LT). The more fit you are, the more you'll be able to push your pace above that LT. It's not uncommon for elite athletes to time trial at 10 to 15% above their LT. Amateur athletes will more likely time trial just at the LT or just a hair above. Experiment with this brisk pace in training to get a good feel for your body and just how long you can hold this pace.

Since time trialing is a race against the clock, you're looking to blast out of the start line and post the best time you possibly can. A proper warm-up is critical. When attempting to hit your TT pace as soon as possible, you will undoubtedly increase the amount of lactic acid in the body. A proper warm-up prepares the body for this, allowing you to settle into your TT pace early in the ride. Without a proper warm-up, your lactic acid levels will spike, causing you to immediately slow your pace and recover from the leg burning and rapid breathing that come with it. Many riders bring their trainers to a TT race so they can warm up near the start line. Here's what a quality thirty- to forty-minute warm-up looks like:

Minutes	Pace
5:00	Easy
3:00	Cruising
2:00	Steady
3:00	Cruising
2:00	Steady
3:00	Cruising
2:00	Brisk
3:00	Easy
2:00	Brisk
3:00	Easy
0:45	Max
3:00	Easy
0:45	Max
5:00	Easy

Coming off your warm-up, your goal is to get to the start line within five to ten minutes of completion. This isn't always a possibility due to event staging protocols, but do the best you can with the timing of your warm-up. While it may seem counterintuitive to do maximal efforts at the tail end of your warm-up, this is the crucial piece of the puzzle. Tapping into that VO2 energy system allows your body to produce lactic acid at an accelerated rate and get yourself ready for the effort to come. You're priming the pump, so to speak, readying the body for that start line burst and quick acceleration into your race pace. Don't forget to practice your warm-up as part of your training.

A 40K is a long haul. If you were to plot out your effort, it should look like a short stair step to race pace, followed by a long sustainable effort, concluding with a final stair-step finish-line kick. Picture it like this:

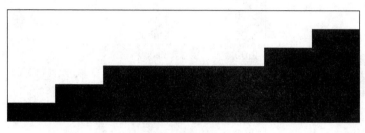

Ideal TT effort graph

The mistake of many beginners is to go out too hard, blow up, recover slightly, and gradually build to the finish.

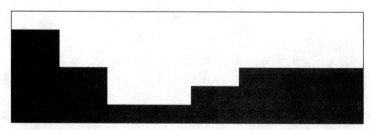

Too-quick start, blow-up, sustainable finish

Another relatively common novice mistake is starting off very conservatively, taking too much time to find a solid racing pace (this usually happens when you haven't practiced pacing enough). Racing like this leaves you crossing the finish line feeling like you could have gone harder. Ideally, you should cross the finish line feeling like you left absolutely everything you had on the course.

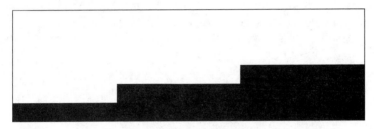

Never hitting a true race pace

POSITIONING

One of the most critical aspects of time trialing, second only to training, is your position on the bike. Since wind resistance provides the greatest form of drag to a cyclist, you need to shoot for the most aerodynamically comfortable position possible. That's not to say you should contort yourself to the point of discomfort. A highly aerodynamic position that is going to make your back, neck, or hamstrings seize after thirty minutes is obviously not going to get you very far. You also don't want to get so aero you can't produce enough power to go fast. Too extreme of a position can limit the range of motion in your hips and legs. You should feel like you can pedal freely and powerfully.

Likewise, you need to be able to steer. If you drop your bars too low, you may find that you can't handle the bike safely at speed. Gradually lower your aerobars and bring the elbows in to a position that is tolerable for the duration of your 40K effort and still allows safe steering.

THE 40K TT PLAN AT A GLANCE

As you might expect, this plan, because it's designed for racers, is more intense than the previous two. It also includes a new element—the RBI, or rest between intervals, on days when you are performing max efforts. Since you are training your body to push very hard and recover quickly before pushing again, it's important to pay more attention to the recovery period between interval efforts.

WEEKS 1–4

WEEK	Monday	Tuesday	Wednesday	Thursday	Friday	Saturday	Sunday
1	Rest day	1:30 Cruising + 3 × 10 min. Steady	1:00 Cruising on TT bike (get comfortable with TT position)	1:30 Cruising + 4 × 6 min. Brisk	0:30 Easy	3:00 Cruising + 3 × 20 min. Steady/Brisk (15 min. Steady/5 min. Brisk)	2:00 Cruising
2	Rest day	1:30 Cruising + 2 × 15 min. Steady	1:15 Cruising on TT bike (focus on TT position)	1:30 Cruising + 3 × 8 min. Brisk	0:45 Easy	3:00 Cruising + 2 × 30 min. Steady/Brisk (20 min. Steady/10 min. Brisk)	2:15 Cruising
3	Rest day	1:30 Cruising + 2 × 20 min. Steady on TT bike	1:45 Cruising	1:30 Cruising + 3 × 10 min. Brisk on TT bike	0:45 Easy	3:00 Cruising + 4 × 15 min. Brisk/Max (12 min. Brisk/3 min. Max with 10 min. RBI)	2:30 Cruising
4	Rest day	1:15 Cruising	1:00 Easy	1:15 Cruising	Rest day	2:00 Cruising	1:30 Cruising

WEEKS 5–8

W E E K	Mon- day	Tuesday	Wednes- day	Thursday	Friday	Saturday	Sunday
5	Rest day	1:30 Cruising + 1 × 30 min. Steady on TT bike	1:15 Cruising	1:30 Cruising +5 × 5 min. Max on TT bike with 5 min. RBI	0:45 Easy	3:00 Cruising +3 × 20 min. Brisk/ Max (15 min. Brisk/ 5 min. Max with 10–15 min. RBI)	2:15 Cruising
6	Rest day	1:30 Cruising +1 × 40 min. Steady on TT bike	1:45 Cruising	1:30 Cruising +4 × 6 min. Max on TT bike with 5 min. RBI	0:45 Easy	3:00 Cruising +2 × 30 min. Brisk on TT bike	2:30 Cruising
7	Rest day	1:30 Cruising +1 × 45 min. Steady on TT bike	2:00 Cruising	1:30 Cruising +5 × 6 min. Max on TT bike with 4 min. RBI	Rest day (taper begins)	2:00 Cruising	1:30 Cruising +5 × 3 min. Max on TT bike with 5–6 min. RBI
8	Rest day (taper- ing)	1:30 Cruising +4 × 5 min. Brisk on TT bike	0:45 Easy	1:00 Cruising +4 × 5 min. Steady/Max (4 min. Steady/1 min. Max with 10 min. RBI)	0:30 Easy or rest day	1:15 Cruising+ 4 × 3 min. Brisk/Max on TT bike (2 min. Brisk/ 1 min. Max with 10 min. RBI)	**40K TT Event!**

40K TT PLAN WEEK BY WEEK

Here is a detailed breakdown of what you should be doing on each day. If you have a heart rate monitor, you can photocopy these pages and write your personal heart rate numbers next to each entry.

40K TT	WEEK 1, DAY 1
Goal for the day: Rest	
Plan for the day: Rest day	

40K TT					WEEK 1, DAY 2
Length: 1 hour, 30 minutes					
Goal for the day: Hard					
Plan for the day: Cruising pace with 3 separate 10-minute intervals at Steady pace					
Time	Time elapse	Pace	Perceived Effort	% of Max	Your Heart Rate Target (fill in)
0–15	15	Cruising	3–4	65–74%	
15–25	10	Steady	5–6	75–84%	
25–35	10	Cruising	3–4	65–74%	
35–45	10	Steady	5–6	75–84%	
45–55	10	Cruising	3–4	65–74%	
55–1:05	10	Steady	5–6	75–84%	
1:05–1:30	25	Cruising	3–4	65–74%	

40K TT					WEEK 1, DAY 3
Length: 1 hour					
Goal for the day: Easy					
Plan for the day: Cruising pace					
Tip: Use your TT bike or aerobars to become comfortable with TT position					
Time	Time elapse	Pace	Perceived Effort	% of Max	Your Heart Rate Target (fill in)
0–60	60	Cruising	3–4	65–74%	

40K TT					WEEK 1, DAY 4
Length: 1 hour, 30 minutes					
Goal for the day: Hard					
Plan for the day: Cruising pace with 4 separate 6-minute intervals at Brisk pace					
Time	Time elapse	Pace	Perceived Effort	% of Max	Your Heart Rate Target (fill in)
0–15	15	Cruising	3–4	65–74%	
15–21	6	Brisk	7–8	85–94%	
21–27	6	Cruising	3–4	65–74%	
27–33	6	Brisk	7–8	85–94%	
33–39	6	Cruising	3–4	65–74%	
39–45	6	Brisk	7–8	85–94%	
45–51	6	Cruising	3–4	65–74%	
51–57	6	Brisk	7–8	85–94%	
57–1:30	33	Cruising	3–4	65–74%	

40K TT					WEEK 1, DAY 5

Length: 30 minutes

Goal for the day: Easy

Plan for the day: Easy pace

Time	Time elapse	Pace	Perceived Effort	% of Max	Your Heart Rate Target (fill in)
0–30	30	Easy	1–2	60–64%	

40K TT					WEEK 1, DAY 6

Length: 3 hours

Goal for the day: Hard

Plan for the day: Cruising pace with 3 separate 20-minute intervals at Steady/Brisk pace (15 minutes at Steady and 5 minutes at Brisk for each interval)

Time	Time elapse	Pace	Perceived Effort	% of Max	Your Heart Rate Target (fill in)
0–30	30	Cruising	3–4	65–74%	
30–45	15	Steady	5–6	75–84%	
45–50	5	Brisk	7–8	85–94%	
50–1:05	15	Cruising	3–4	65–74%	
1:05–1:20	15	Steady	5–6	75–84%	
1:20–1:25	5	Brisk	7–8	85–94%	
1:25–1:40	15	Cruising	3–4	65–74%	
1:40–1:55	15	Steady	5–6	75–84%	
1:55–2:00	5	Brisk	7–8	85–94%	
2:00–3:00	1:00	Cruising	3–4	65–74%	

40K TT					WEEK 1, DAY 7
Length: 2 hours					
Goal for the day: Long					
Plan for the day: Cruising pace					
Time	Time elapse	Pace	Perceived Effort	% of Max	Your Heart Rate Target (fill in)
0–2:00	2:00	Cruising	3–4	65–74%	

40K TT	WEEK 2, DAY 1
Goal for the day: Rest	
Plan for the day: Rest day	

40K TT					WEEK 2, DAY 2
Length: 1 hour, 30 minutes					
Goal for the day: Hard					
Plan for the day: Cruising pace with 2 separate 15-minute intervals at Steady pace					
Time	Time elapse	Pace	Perceived Effort	% of Max	Your Heart Rate Target (fill in)
0–15	15	Cruising	3–4	65–74%	
15–30	15	Steady	5–6	75–84%	
30–40	10	Cruising	3–4	65–74%	
40–55	15	Steady	5–6	75–84%	
55–1:30	35	Cruising	3–4	65–74%	

40K TT					WEEK 2, DAY 3
Length: 1 hour, 15 minutes					
Goal for the day: Easy					
Plan for the day: Cruising pace					
Tip: Use your TT bike or aerobars to become comfortable with TT position					
Time	**Time elapse**	**Pace**	**Perceived Effort**	**% of Max**	**Your Heart Rate Target (fill in)**
0–1:15	1:15	Cruising	3–4	65–74%	

40K TT					WEEK 2, DAY 4
Length: 1 hour, 30 minutes					
Goal for the day: Hard					
Plan for the day: Cruising pace with 3 separate 8-minute intervals at Brisk pace					
Time	**Time elapse**	**Pace**	**Perceived Effort**	**% of Max**	**Your Heart Rate Target (fill in)**
0–20	20	Cruising	3–4	65–74%	
20–28	8	Brisk	7–8	85–94%	
28–33	5	Cruising	3–4	65–74%	
33–41	8	Brisk	7–8	85–94%	
41–46	5	Cruising	3–4	65–74%	
46–54	8	Brisk	7–8	85–94%	
54–1:30	36	Cruising	3–4	65–74%	

40K TT					WEEK 2, DAY 5
Length: 45 minutes					
Goal for the day: Easy					
Plan for the day: Easy pace					
Time	Time elapse	Pace	Perceived Effort	% of Max	Your Heart Rate Target (fill in)
0–45	45	Easy	1–2	60–64%	

40K TT					WEEK 2, DAY 6
Length: 3 hours					
Goal for the day: Hard					
Plan for the day: Cruising pace with 2 separate 30-minute intervals at Steady/ Brisk pace (20 minutes at Steady and 10 minutes at Brisk for each interval)					
Time	Time elapse	Pace	Perceived Effort	% of Max	Your Heart Rate Target (fill in)
0–30	30	Cruising	3–4	65–74%	
30–50	20	Steady	5–6	75–84%	
50–60	10	Brisk	7–8	85–94%	
60–1:15	15	Cruising	3–4	65–74%	
1:15–1:35	20	Steady	5–6	75–84%	
1:35–1:45	10	Brisk	7–8	85–94%	
1:45–3:00	1:15	Cruising	3–4	65–74%	

40K TT					WEEK 2, DAY 7
Length: 2 hours, 15 minutes					
Goal for the day: Long					
Plan for the day: Cruising pace					
Time	Time elapse	Pace	Perceived Effort	% of Max	Your Heart Rate Target (fill in)
0–2:15	2:15	Cruising	3–4	65–74%	

40K TT	WEEK 3, DAY 1
Goal for the day: Rest	
Plan for the day: Rest day	

40K TT					WEEK 3, DAY 2
Length: 1 hour, 30 minutes					
Goal for the day: Hard					
Plan for the day: Cruising pace with 2 separate 20-minute intervals at Steady pace					
Tip: Use your TT bike or aerobars to become comfortable with TT position					
Time	Time elapse	Pace	Perceived Effort	% of Max	Your Heart Rate Target (fill in)
0–15	15	Cruising	3–4	65–74%	
15–35	20	Steady	5–6	75–84%	
35–45	10	Cruising	3–4	65–74%	
45–1:05	20	Steady	5–6	75–84%	
1:05–1:30	25	Cruising	3–4	65–74%	

40K TT					WEEK 3, DAY 3
Length: 1 hour, 45 minutes					
Goal for the day: Easy					
Plan for the day: Cruising pace					
Time	Time elapse	Pace	Perceived Effort	% of Max	Your Heart Rate Target (fill in)
0–1:45	1:45	Cruising	3–4	65–74%	

40K TT					WEEK 3, DAY 4
Length: 1 hour, 30 minutes					
Goal for the day: Hard					
Plan for the day: Cruising pace with 3 separate 10-minute intervals at Brisk pace					
Tip: Use your TT bike or aerobars to become comfortable with TT position					
Time	Time elapse	Pace	Perceived Effort	% of Max	Your Heart Rate Target (fill in)
0–20	20	Cruising	3–4	65–74%	
20–30	10	Brisk	7–8	85–94%	
30–40	10	Cruising	3–4	65–74%	
40–50	10	Brisk	7–8	85–94%	
50–60	10	Cruising	3–4	65–74%	
60–1:10	10	Brisk	7–8	85–94%	
1:10–1:30	20	Cruising	3–4	65–74%	

40K TT					WEEK 3, DAY 5
Length: 45 minutes					
Goal for the day: Easy					
Plan for the day: Easy pace					
Time	Time elapse	Pace	Perceived Effort	% of Max	Your Heart Rate Target (fill in)
0–45	45	Easy	1–2	60–64%	

40K TT					WEEK 3, DAY 6
Length: 3 hours					
Goal for the day: Hard					
Plan for the day: Cruising pace with 4 separate 15-minute intervals at Brisk/ Max pace (12 minutes at Brisk and 3 minutes at Max for each interval); rest for 10 minutes at Easy pace between intervals					
Time	Time elapse	Pace	Perceived Effort	% of Max	Your Heart Rate Target (fill in)
0–45	45	Cruising	3–4	65–74%	
45–57	12	Brisk	7–8	85–94%	
57–60	3	Max	9–10	95–100%	
60–1:10	10	Easy	1–2	60–64%	
1:10–1:22	12	Brisk	7–8	85–94%	
1:22–1:25	3	Max	9–10	95–100%	
1:25–1:35	10	Easy	1–2	60–64%	
1:35–1:47	12	Brisk	7–8	85–94%	
1:47–1:50	3	Max	9–10	95–100%	
1:50–2:00	10	Easy	1–2	60–64%	
2:00–2:12	12	Brisk	7–8	85–94%	
2:12–2:15	3	Max	9–10	95–100%	
2:15–3:00	45	Cruising	3–4	65–74%	

40K TT					WEEK 3, DAY 7
Length: 2 hours, 30 minutes					
Goal for the day: Long					
Plan for the day: Cruising pace					
Time	**Time elapse**	**Pace**	**Perceived Effort**	**% of Max**	**Your Heart Rate Target (fill in)**
0–2:30	2:30	Cruising	3–4	65–74%	

40K TT	WEEK 4, DAY 1
Goal for the day: Rest	
Plan for the day: Rest day	

40K TT					WEEK 4, DAY 2
Length: 1 hour, 15 minutes					
Goal for the day: Easy					
Plan for the day: Cruising pace					
Time	**Time elapse**	**Pace**	**Perceived Effort**	**% of Max**	**Your Heart Rate Target (fill in)**
0–1:15	1:15	Cruising	3–4	65–74%	

40K TT					WEEK 4, DAY 3
Length: 1 hour					
Goal for the day: Easy					
Plan for the day: Easy pace					
Time	**Time elapse**	**Pace**	**Perceived Effort**	**% of Max**	**Your Heart Rate Target (fill in)**
0–1:00	1:00	Easy	1–2	60–64%	

40K TT					WEEK 4, DAY 4
Length: 1 hour, 15 minutes					
Goal for the day: Easy					
Plan for the day: Cruising pace					
Time	**Time elapse**	**Pace**	**Perceived Effort**	**% of Max**	**Your Heart Rate Target (fill in)**
0–1:15	1:15	Cruising	3–4	65–74%	

40K TT	WEEK 4, DAY 5
Goal for the day: Rest	
Plan for the day: Rest day	

40K TT					WEEK 4, DAY 6
Length: 1 hour, 30 minutes					
Goal for the day: Long					
Plan for the day: Cruising pace					
Time	Time elapse	Pace	Perceived Effort	% of Max	Your Heart Rate Target (fill in)
0–1:30	1:30	Cruising	3–4	65–74%	

40K TT					WEEK 4, DAY 7
Length: 2 hours					
Goal for the day: Long					
Plan for the day: Cruising pace					
Time	Time elapse	Pace	Perceived Effort	% of Max	Your Heart Rate Target (fill in)
0–2:00	2:00	Cruising	3–4	65–74%	

40K TT	WEEK 5, DAY 1
Goal for the day: Rest	
Plan for the day: Rest day	

40K TT					WEEK 5, DAY 2
Length: 1 hour, 30 minutes					
Goal for the day: Hard					
Plan for the day: Cruising pace with 1 separate 30-minute interval at Steady pace					
Tip: Use your TT bike or aerobars to become comfortable with TT position					
Time	**Time elapse**	**Pace**	**Perceived Effort**	**% of Max**	**Your Heart Rate Target (fill in)**
0–30	30	Cruising	3–4	65–74%	
30–60	30	Steady	5–6	75–84%	
60–1:30	30	Cruising	3–4	65–74%	

40K TT					WEEK 5, DAY 3
Length: 1 hour, 15 minutes					
Goal for the day: Easy					
Plan for the day: Cruising pace					
Time	**Time elapse**	**Pace**	**Perceived Effort**	**% of Max**	**Your Heart Rate Target (fill in)**
0–1:15	1:15	Cruising	3–4	65–74%	

40K TT					WEEK 5, DAY 4
Length: 1 hour, 30 minutes					
Goal for the day: Hard					
Plan for the day: Cruising pace with 5 separate 5-minute intervals at Max pace; rest for 5 minutes at Easy pace between intervals					
Tip: Use your TT bike or aerobars to become comfortable with TT position					
Time	Time elapse	Pace	Perceived Effort	% of Max	Your Heart Rate Target (fill in)
0–20	20	Cruising	3–4	65–74%	
20–25	5	Max	9–10	95–100%	
25–30	5	Easy	1–2	60–64%	
30–35	5	Max	9–10	95–100%	
35–40	5	Easy	1–2	60–64%	
40–45	5	Max	9–10	95–100%	
45–50	5	Easy	1–2	60–64%	
50–55	5	Max	9–10	95–100%	
55–60	5	Easy	1–2	60–64%	
60–1:05	5	Max	9–10	95–100%	
1:05–1:10	5	Easy	1–2	60–64%	
1:10–1:30	20	Cruising	3–4	65–74%	

40K TT					WEEK 5, DAY 5
Length: 45 minutes					
Goal for the day: Easy					
Plan for the day: Easy pace					
Time	Time elapse	Pace	Perceived Effort	% of Max	Your Heart Rate Target (fill in)
0–45	45	Easy	1–2	60–64%	

40K TT					WEEK 5, DAY 6
Length: 3 hours					
Goal for the day: Hard					
Plan for the day: Cruising pace with 3 separate 20-minute intervals at Brisk/ Max pace (15 minutes at Brisk and 5 minutes at Max for each interval); rest for 10 to 15 minutes at Easy pace between intervals					
Time	**Time elapse**	**Pace**	**Perceived Effort**	**% of Max**	**Your Heart Rate Target (fill in)**
0–45	45	Cruising	3–4	65–74%	
45–60	15	Brisk	7–8	85–94%	
60–1:05	5	Max	9–10	95–100%	
1:05–1:15	10	Easy	1–2	60–64%	
1:15–1:30	15	Brisk	7–8	85–94%	
1:30–1:35	5	Max	9–10	95–100%	
1:35–1:45	10	Easy	1–2	60–64%	
1:45–2:00	15	Brisk	7–8	85–94%	
2:00–2:05	5	Max	9–10	95–100%	
2:05–2:15	10	Easy	1–2	60–64%	
2:15–3:00	45	Cruising	3–4	65–74%	

40K TT					WEEK 5, DAY 7
Length: 2 hours, 15 minutes					
Goal for the day: Long					
Plan for the day: Cruising pace					
Time	**Time elapse**	**Pace**	**Perceived Effort**	**% of Max**	**Your Heart Rate Target (fill in)**
0–2:15	2:15	Cruising	3–4	65–74%	

40K TT				WEEK 6, DAY 1	
Goal for the day: Rest					
Plan for the day: Rest day					

40K TT				WEEK 6, DAY 2	
Length: 1 hour, 30 minutes					
Goal for the day: Hard					
Plan for the day: Cruising pace with 1 separate 40-minute interval at Steady pace					
Tip: Use your TT bike or aerobars to become comfortable with TT position					
Time	Time elapse	Pace	Perceived Effort	% of Max	Your Heart Rate Target (fill in)
0–20	20	Cruising	3–4	65–74%	
20–60	40	Steady	5–6	75–84%	
60–1:30	30	Cruising	3–4	65–74%	

40K TT				WEEK 6, DAY 3	
Length: 1 hour, 45 minutes					
Goal for the day: Long					
Plan for the day: Cruising pace					
Time	Time elapse	Pace	Perceived Effort	% of Max	Your Heart Rate Target (fill in)
0–1:45	1:45	Cruising	3–4	65–74%	

40K TT					WEEK 6, DAY 4

Length: 1 hour, 30 minutes

Goal for the day: Hard

Plan for the day: Cruising pace with 4 separate 6-minute intervals at Max pace; rest for 5 minutes at Easy pace between intervals

Tip: Use your TT bike or aerobars to become comfortable with TT position

Time	Time elapse	Pace	Perceived Effort	% of Max	Your Heart Rate Target (fill in)
0–20	20	Cruising	3–4	65–74%	
20–26	6	Max	9–10	95–100%	
26–31	5	Easy	1–2	60–64%	
31–37	6	Max	9–10	95–100%	
37–42	5	Easy	1–2	60–64%	
42–48	6	Max	9–10	95–100%	
48–53	5	Easy	1–2	60–64%	
53–59	6	Max	9–10	95–100%	
59–1:04	5	Easy	1–2	60–64%	
1:04–1:30	26	Cruising	3–4	65–74%	

40K TT					WEEK 6, DAY 5

Length: 45 minutes

Goal for the day: Easy

Plan for the day: Easy pace

Time	Time elapse	Pace	Perceived Effort	% of Max	Your Heart Rate Target (fill in)
0–45	45	Easy	1–2	60–64%	

40K TT					WEEK 6, DAY 6
Length: 3 hours					
Goal for the day: Hard					
Plan for the day: Cruising pace with 2 separate 30-minute intervals at Brisk pace					
Tip: Use your TT bike or aerobars to become comfortable with TT position					
Time	Time elapse	Pace	Perceived Effort	% of Max	Your Heart Rate Target (fill in)
0–30	30	Cruising	3–4	65–74%	
30–60	30	Brisk	7–8	85–94%	
60–1:15	15	Cruising	3–4	65–74%	
1:15–1:45	30	Brisk	7–8	85–94%	
1:45–3:00	1:15	Cruising	3–4	65–74%	

40K TT					WEEK 6, DAY 7
Length: 2 hours, 30 minutes					
Goal for the day: Long					
Plan for the day: Cruising pace					
Time	Time elapse	Pace	Perceived Effort	% of Max	Your Heart Rate Target (fill in)
0–2:30	2:30	Cruising	3–4	65–74%	

40K TT	WEEK 7, DAY 1
Goal for the day: Rest	
Plan for the day: Rest day	

40K TT					WEEK 7, DAY 2

Length: 1 hour, 30 minutes

Goal for the day: Hard

Plan for the day: Cruising pace with 1 separate 45-minute interval at Steady pace

Tip: Use your TT bike or aerobars to become comfortable with TT position

Time	Time elapse	Pace	Perceived Effort	% of Max	Your Heart Rate Target (fill in)
0–15	15	Cruising	3–4	65–74%	
15–60	45	Steady	5–6	75–84%	
60–1:30	30	Cruising	3–4	65–74%	

40K TT					WEEK 7, DAY 3

Length: 2 hours

Goal for the day: Long

Plan for the day: Cruising pace

Time	Time elapse	Pace	Perceived Effort	% of Max	Your Heart Rate Target (fill in)
0–2:00	2:00	Cruising	3–4	65–74%	

40K TT					WEEK 7, DAY 4
Length: 1 hour, 30 minutes					
Goal for the day: Hard					
Plan for the day: Cruising pace with 5 separate 6-minute intervals at Max pace; rest for 4 minutes at Easy pace between intervals					
Tip: Use your TT bike or aerobars to become comfortable with TT position					
Time	**Time elapse**	**Pace**	**Perceived Effort**	**% of Max**	**Your Heart Rate Target (fill in)**
0–20	20	Cruising	3–4	65–74%	
20–26	6	Max	9–10	95–100%	
26–30	4	Easy	1–2	60–64%	
30–36	6	Max	9–10	95–100%	
36–40	4	Easy	1–2	60–64%	
40–46	6	Max	9–10	95–100%	
46–50	4	Easy	1–2	60–64%	
50–56	6	Max	9–10	95–100%	
56–60	4	Easy	1–2	60–64%	
60–1:06	6	Max	9–10	95–100%	
1:06–1:10	4	Easy	1–2	60–64%	
1:10–1:30	20	Cruising	3–4	65–74%	

40K TT	WEEK 7, DAY 5
Goal for the day: Rest	
Plan for the day: Rest day (taper begins)	

40K TT					WEEK 7, DAY 6
Length: 2 hours					
Goal for the day: Long					
Plan for the day: Cruising pace					
Time	Time elapse	Pace	Perceived Effort	% of Max	Your Heart Rate Target (fill in)
0–2:00	2:00	Cruising	3–4	65–74%	

40K TT					WEEK 7, DAY 7
Length: 1 hour, 30 minutes					
Goal for the day: Hard					
Plan for the day: Cruising pace with 5 separate 3-minute intervals at Max pace; rest for 5 to 6 minutes at Easy pace between intervals					
Tip: Use your TT bike or aerobars to become comfortable with TT position					
Time	Time elapse	Pace	Perceived Effort	% of Max	Your Heart Rate Target (fill in)
0–20	20	Cruising	3–4	65–74%	
20–23	3	Max	9–10	95–100%	
23–28	5	Easy	1–2	60–64%	
28–31	3	Max	9–10	95–100%	
31–36	5	Easy	1–2	60–64%	
36–39	3	Max	9–10	95–100%	
39–44	5	Easy	1–2	60–64%	
44–47	3	Max	9–10	95–100%	
47–52	5	Easy	1–2	60–64%	
52–55	3	Max	9–10	95–100%	
55–60	5	Easy	1–2	60–64%	
60–1:30	30	Cruising	3–4	65–74%	

40K TT					WEEK 8, DAY 1
Goal for the day: Rest					
Plan for the day: Rest day (tapering)					

40K TT					WEEK 8, DAY 2
Length: 1 hour, 30 minutes					
Goal for the day: Hard					
Plan for the day: Cruising pace with 4 separate 5-minute intervals at Brisk pace					
Tip: Use your TT bike or aerobars to become comfortable with TT position					
Time	Time elapse	Pace	Perceived Effort	% of Max	Your Heart Rate Target (fill in)
0–15	15	Cruising	3–4	65–74%	
15–20	5	Brisk	7–8	85–94%	
20–30	10	Cruising	3–4	65–74%	
30–35	5	Brisk	7–8	85–94%	
35–45	10	Cruising	3–4	65–74%	
45–50	5	Brisk	7–8	85–94%	
50–60	10	Cruising	3–4	65–74%	
60–1:05	5	Brisk	7–8	85–94%	
1:05–1:30	25	Cruising	3–4	65–74%	

40K TT					WEEK 8, DAY 3
Length: 45 minutes					
Goal for the day: Easy					
Plan for the day: Easy pace					
Time	Time elapse	Pace	Perceived Effort	% of Max	Your Heart Rate Target (fill in)
0–45	45	Easy	1–2	60–64%	

40K TT					WEEK 8, DAY 4
Length: 1 hour					
Goal for the day: Hard					
Plan for the day: Cruising pace with 4 separate 5-minute intervals at Steady/ Max pace (4 minutes at Steady and 1 minute at Max for each interval); rest for 10 minutes at Easy pace between intervals					
Time	Time elapse	Pace	Perceived Effort	% of Max	Your Heart Rate Target (fill in)
0–5	5	Cruising	3–4	65–74%	
5–9	4	Steady	5–6	75–84%	
9–10	1	Max	9–10	95–100%	
10–20	10	Easy	1–2	60–64%	
20–24	4	Steady	5–6	75–84%	
24–25	1	Max	9–10	95–100%	
25–35	10	Easy	1–2	60–64%	
35–39	4	Steady	5–6	75–84%	
39–40	1	Max	9–10	95–100%	
40–50	10	Easy	1–2	60–64%	
50–54	4	Steady	5–6	75–84%	
54–55	1	Max	9–10	95–100%	
55–60	5	Easy	1–2	60–64%	

40K TT					WEEK 8, DAY 5
Length: 30 minutes (or rest day)					
Goal for the day: Easy					
Plan for the day: Easy pace					
Time	Time elapse	Pace	Perceived Effort	% of Max	Your Heart Rate Target (fill in)
0–30	30	Easy	1–2	60–64%	

40K TT					WEEK 8, DAY 6
Length: 1 hour, 15 minutes					
Goal for the day: Hard					
Plan for the day: Cruising pace with 4 separate 3-minute intervals at Brisk/Max pace (2 minutes at Brisk and 1 minute at Max for each interval); rest for 10 minutes at Easy pace between intervals					
Tip: Use your TT bike or aerobars to become comfortable with TT position					
Time	**Time elapse**	**Pace**	**Perceived Effort**	**% of Max**	**Your Heart Rate Target (fill in)**
0–10	10	Cruising	3–4	65–74%	
10–12	2	Brisk	7–8	85–94%	
12–13	1	Max	9–10	95–100%	
13–23	10	Easy	1–2	60–64%	
23–25	2	Brisk	7–8	85–94%	
25–26	1	Max	9–10	95–100%	
26–36	10	Easy	1–2	60–64%	
36–38	2	Brisk	7–8	85–94%	
38–39	1	Max	9–10	95–100%	
39–49	10	Easy	1–2	60–64%	
49–51	2	Brisk	7–8	85–94%	
51–52	1	Max	9–10	95–100%	
52–1:15	23	Easy	1–2	60–64%	

40K TT EVENT!	WEEK 8, DAY 7

BUYING SPEED

Once you get into TT, you'll be looking for every little advantage to help you go just that much faster. The easiest way to get faster is reducing aerodynamic drag, so air flows as smoothly as possible over you. Cyclists have gone to incredible extremes to become more aero. Taping down zippers, removing any unnecessary equipment from the bike (such as saddlebags and pumps), cutting brake and derailleur cables shorter, and extreme haircuts are all part of the game. As comical as it may sound, a few women have been known to tape down their breasts in hopes of creating a more aerodynamic form. A few special items of gear can help as well:

Aerobars

If you don't have a TT-specific bike, aerodynamic handlebars are the single-best piece of equipment you can invest in. These forearm-supported bars allow you to lie forward in an attempt to flatten out your back and allow air to move over your head as opposed to smacking you in the chest. Bars are available in various sizes and adjustable to the width of a rider's chest and arm reach.

Time trial helmet

The teardrop shape of a time trial–specific helmet allows air to travel in a more uninterrupted fashion across the head and down the spine.

Skinsuit

A skinsuit is a snug-fitting singlet, jersey and shorts in one, with a thin zipper. A form-fitting top means no unnecessary wrinkles and bunching material flapping in the wind and slowing you down.

Shoe covers

Lightweight Lycra or plastic slip-on shoe covers will make certain the air flows smoothly over the Velcro straps or buckles that secure your cycling shoes.

OFF-SEASON AND SUPPLEMENTAL TRAINING

Some people ride year round, but I'm of the school of thought that you really shouldn't. Everyone, even the pros, needs a mental, if not physical, break from the bike to explore other interests and do some other types of exercise for balanced fitness.

This type of cross training is especially important for women. Turning pedals trims your thighs and strengthens your heart, but it doesn't build your bones, especially in the spine, hips, and arms, where women are prone to fractures later in life. At the very least, you should do some resistance training two to three times a week in the off-season and one to two times a week during the cycling season to maintain lean muscle mass and keep your skeleton strong.

CROSS TRAINING

Cross training gives you a break from the bike to prevent boredom and provides countless ways to stay fit when you can't ride because of travel or weather. Here are a few cross training activities to try:

Trail running

Most of my cycling friends hate running. Understandably. When you're used to cruising at 16 MPH and coasting down hills, the constant plodding on the pavement feels more like work than play. Plus, running doesn't really complement cycling (it's powered by your hamstrings, not your quads), so it won't necessarily make you faster on your bike. That's why I love trail running. Running on dirt paths or hiking trails is nearly as fun as riding and provides cycling-specific fitness benefits. Traipsing up hills works your quads and improves your pedaling power. It burns about ten calories a minute, so a twenty-five- or thirty-minute jog is all you need to get in a good workout. And it strengthens your bones and connective tissues. Just remember to stretch afterward. Running makes your muscles feel tight.

Swimming

Slicing through the water takes your curled-up cycling body and stretches it out long and lean. It develops the core and upper body muscles that cycling neglects. And it's an amazing cardiovascular workout. Swimming won't build your bones, however, so be sure to mix it up with resistance training.

Step aerobics

Any kind of aerobics class will help keep your heart and lungs fit, but step aerobics is best if you're looking for an on-the-bike benefit. Springing up and down off the step uses the same muscles as pedaling, so you'll have more snap in sprints and climbs. It also burns more calories than other aerobic class workouts.

Circuit training

Circuit training is a style of resistance training in which you jump from one exercise to the next with no rest in between. Lifting like this keeps your heart rate up, so you get a cardiovascular benefit while you strengthen your muscles. People who get bored in the gym like circuit training because it eliminates all the sitting around between sets. For the best results, set up your circuit so you alternate between upper and lower body moves—e.g., squat, chest press, lunge, bent-over row, and so on. Most circuits include about eight exercises that you cycle through two to three times.

Snow sports

Cross-country skiing and snowshoeing are outstanding activities for snowbound cyclists because they're aerobically demanding and tap into many of the same muscles as cycling. If you live somewhere the snow flies two or three (or more . . .) months a year, they're the perfect way to burn tons of calories and stay fit to ride come spring.

Yoga/Pilates

Neither yoga nor Pilates is particularly aerobic, so they won't keep you cardiovascularly fit, but they stretch you out and strengthen your core so you feel better on your bike. I recommend incorporating at least a few moves from each (e.g., downward-facing dog from yoga, the hundred from Pilates) into your routine year-round.

TAKE IT INSIDE

As the off-season wanes, you'll likely find that you're ready to get back on your bike before the weather is fully ready to cooperate. That's why I have my beloved indoor trainer set up in my laundry room next to a picture window with an iPod sound system nearby. It can be 42 degrees and sleeting and I can still be happily humming along on my road bike.

Of course, I'd *much* rather be outside in the fresh air; I've been known to ride in sub-20-degree temperatures. But there are some distinct advantages to indoor cycling that can make it a smart train-

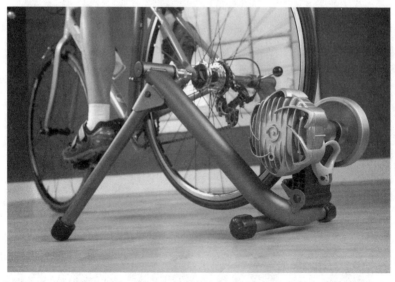

When you just can't get outside to ride, a turbo trainer provides an alternative way to spin your wheels.

ing option year-round, especially as you're ramping back up in the off-season. For one, trainers allow for consistency. You can do six three-minute intervals on your trainer and know that the conditions will be exactly the same each time. There's no traffic or stop signs to interrupt a workout. And it's quick. Just throw on your clothes and hop aboard; there's no hunting for gloves, vest, booties, spare tubes, or other accessories.

Types of trainers

Below are a few popular options for indoor bike trainers:

- **Turbo trainers:** Known simply as "trainers," these triangular platforms fasten onto your rear wheel, which rolls along on a metal drum that provides resistance much like riding outdoors. Prices range from around $100 to around $500, and you really do get what you pay for. Higher-end models are whisper quiet and extremely smooth and stable.

- **Rollers:** As the name implies, this type of trainer is nothing more than a set of steel drums on a rectangular frame. You place your bike on top, hold on to a wall to get balanced, and away you go! Because you have to balance your bike, rollers force you to pedal smoothly and are great for perfecting your pedal stroke. The biggest downside to rollers is you can't get out of the saddle to stand on your pedals to simulate climbing or sprinting without risking flying off the platform and sailing across the room (or just plummeting to the floor). One exception: Inside Ride E-Motion rollers. They're embedded on a sliding platform surrounded by bumpers. They're impossible to ride off and allow you to stand, sprint, and toss the bike around as you would in real riding conditions. This type of technology doesn't come cheap (they run in the $700 range), but if you get serious about year-round riding, they're a good investment.

- **Spinning bikes:** You've likely seen these at the gym, heavy metal behemoths used for Spinning or indoor cycling classes. Most brands offer home models, but they cost from $700 to $2,000 and they take up a lot of space. If you belong to a gym and can get on one regularly, though, they do provide a good cycling-specific workout. You also can take a Spinning class once or twice a week in the off-season to keep your cycling muscles sharp. With any indoor training, it's important to realize that a little goes a long way.

Unlike a real outside ride, you don't coast on your trainer. It's nonstop pedaling action, so an hour is *plenty* of time. Just remember to have a water bottle (and maybe a fan) handy. Without a cooling breeze, you heat up quickly and can feel uncomfortably warm within a few minutes.

Inside trainer workouts

Indoor training can be as simple as hopping on your trainer and pedaling away while watching *Oprah*. But you'll soon find that even with the pop culture distraction, minutes creep by slowly when you're going nowhere fast. Make time fly with these structured workouts. Each one takes less than an hour to complete and is designed to provide a specific fitness benefit.

You can do these workouts two or three times a week during the off-season to keep your cycling muscles sharp and use them as supplemental training year round. They can be done on a Spinning bike in the gym as well as your own personal trainer.

- **Fast Breaks**
  - Warm up for 15 minutes, pedaling at an easy to moderate effort.
  - Click into a gear (or adjust the resistance) so you can pedal at a high cadence of 90 RPM.
  - Accelerate until you are at about 90 to 95% max heart rate (nearly as hard as you can go).
  - Hold that intensity for 2 full minutes.

- Recover 2 minutes at easy pace.
- Repeat 5 times.
- Cool down for 10 minutes.
- Progress to holding each fast break for 3 minutes.
- **Cycling benefit:** Trains your body to use more oxygen to raise your VO2 max.

- **Drop 15s**
  - Warm up for 15 minutes, pedaling at an easy to moderate effort.
  - Click into a fairly large gear (or increase the resistance) that you can't easily spin at a high cadence.
  - Rise out of the saddle and start sprinting.
  - Sit and hold a cadence of about 90 to 110 RPM for 90 seconds (your heart rate should be about 90% max).
  - Downshift and spin easy until you are fully recovered (about 1 to 2 minutes).
  - Repeat the drill for 75 seconds.
  - Continue, dropping interval times by 15 seconds until you hit the final 15-second interval.
  - Cool down for 10 minutes.
  - **Cycling benefit:** Improves top-end power and efficiency.

- **3-2-1s**
  - Warm up for 10 minutes, pedaling at an easy to moderate effort.
  - Increase your intensity to about 80% max heart rate (6 or 7 RPE). Hold it here for 3 minutes.
  - Ramp up the intensity again to about 85% max heart rate (about an 8 RPE). Hold it here for 2 minutes.
  - Crank up the intensity over the final 1 minute so you finish the last 10 to 15 seconds as hard as you can go (10 RPE).
  - Ride easy to fully recover for 10 minutes.

- Repeat the 3-2-1 drill. Ride easy to moderate for the final 10 to 15 minutes.
- Progress to 3 separate 3-2-1 drills (broken up by 10 minutes recovery).
- **Cycling benefit:** Trains your body to repeatedly push and recover on the fly to simulate the rigors of real riding and racing conditions.

- **Triple Tempo**
  - Warm up for 10 minutes, pedaling at an easy to moderate effort.
  - Increase your intensity to 75 to 84% max heart rate. Hold it here for 8 to 10 minutes.
  - Reduce intensity to recover for about 5 minutes.
  - Repeat the "tempo" interval.
  - Pedal at an easy to moderate pace for the final 10 to 15 minutes.
  - Progress to doing 3 tempo intervals with 5 minutes recovery between efforts.
  - **Cycling benefit:** Improves sustainable power, so you can ride longer, more comfortably at higher speeds.

- **Big Gear Endurance**
  - Warm up for 10 minutes.
  - Click into a large gear (or increase the resistance) so you can just pedal about 60 RPM. Hold this effort and intensity for 5 minutes.
  - Recover 5 minutes in an easier gear.
  - Repeat 3 to 4 times.
  - Pedal easy for the final 10 minutes.
  - Work up to doing 2 separate 15-minute intervals with 10 minutes of recovery.
  - **Cycling benefit:** Improves leg strength and power, so

higher intensity rides feel easier. (Skip this drill if you have a history of knee problems.)

- **Hill Surges (prop the front tire on a book to simulate an incline)**
  - Warm up for 10 to 15 minutes at an easy to moderate pace.
  - Click into a harder gear (or increase your resistance) so your pedaling cadence is about 70 RPM and you feel like you're climbing. Climb here for 2 minutes.
  - Accelerate to increase your cadence to about 80 RPM. Hold here for 30 seconds.
  - Click into the next-hardest gear, maintaining your cadence for another 30 seconds.
  - Shift one more gear higher, stand, and accelerate for 15 seconds.
  - Downshift and recover for 3 to 5 minutes.
  - Repeat 5 times.
  - Cool down for 5 to 10 minutes.
  - **Cycling benefit:** Acclimates your body to high-intensity, high-resistance efforts so you can conquer all those local climbs.

- **The Ride:** My favorite format for teaching indoor cycling classes is to simply take the group for an imaginary ride. I cue up premixed CDs that include music of varying tempos and away we go, burning down the pancake-flat roads in Kansas, climbing mountains in Montana, sprinting for town signs along the way. It's super easy to do with an iPod. Note: Indoor training is a great time to work on your cadence. When it says go fast, pick up your pedal speed. During slower songs, add resistance to push the pedals harder. Here's a sample format to follow with some of my favorite songs:
  - **Warm-up:** Energetic song to get you moving ("Music" by Madonna)

- **Flat and fast:** High-tempo cruising song to start picking up the pace ("Break on Through" by The Doors)
- **Sustained climb:** Steady, slower rhythm; moderate to hard effort ("Migra" by Santana)
- **Downhill:** High-speed pedaling, fast and furious ("Girls Got Rhythm" by AC/DC)
- **Big gear paceline:** Steady-tempo effort in a moderately hard gear and brisk (about 90 RPM) cadence ("Days Go By" by Dirty Vegas)
- **Cruising:** Easy spinning for a few minutes of recovery ("A Little Less Conversation" by Elvis)
- **Steep climb:** Hard-driving, slow-tempo beat ("Gangsta's Paradise" by Coolio)
- **Flat and fast:** High-tempo song to spin out your legs ("Vertigo" by U2)
- **Sprints to the finish:** High-energy song to finish with 2 to 3 30-second sprints ("Respect" by Pink)
- **Cool down:** Happy cruising music to let your heart rate come down ("No Rain" by Blind Melon)
- **Cycling benefit:** Trains your body to ride like you do outside. And it's fun.

RESISTANCE/STRENGTH TRAINING

For years cyclists (and other endurance athletes) were scared away from strength training by coaches who warned it would bulk them up and slow them down. That may be true if you go in and pump iron two hours a day like a body-builder. But these days most experts agree that a little strength training can make you better on the bike.

For one, pushing pedals takes power—the ability to do lots of work in a short amount of time. You need strength—the ability to move weight (your own, your bike's . . .)—to have power. Resistance training helps make your muscles strong, so you can produce more power on the bike.

Riding a bike also takes more than strong legs (which riding a bike helps build). Your arms support you on your bars. Your core muscles transfer power and provide a platform for your legs to push against. But cycling alone will not strengthen those muscles.

Finally, we all lose lean muscle mass as a natural part of the aging process. Women don't start out with a whole lot to begin with, so we have less to lose. (Ditto for bone mass.) Resistance training is imperative to maintain the muscle that keeps you strong not just for cycling but for daily living.

You don't need to join a gym or buy any fancy equipment. Just your own body weight and a ten-pound pair of dumbbells will do the trick. Do two to three sets of ten to twelve reps of the following moves. During riding season, aim to do resistance training once or twice a week. Do it two to three days in the off-season.

Stationary bicycle (targets abs)

Lie on your back, hands behind your head, knees bent. Lift your feet off the floor so your legs form a 90-degree angle, calves parallel to the ground. Pull your navel to your spine and lift your head and shoulders off the floor.

Curl your right shoulder across your body toward your left knee while extending the right leg. *Do not draw your left knee into your chest.*

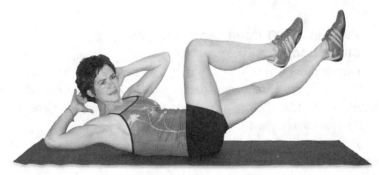

Stationary bicycle curl

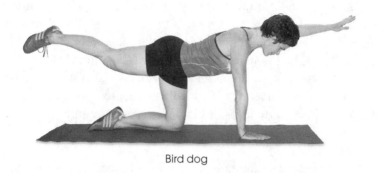

Bird dog

Keeping your torso lifted, switch sides, bringing the right leg back to start and curling your left shoulder toward the right knee, while extending the left leg. That's one rep.

Bird dog (targets back)

Kneel on all fours, with hands directly beneath shoulders and knees directly beneath hips. Keep back straight and head in line with spine.

Simultaneously raise right arm and left leg, extending them in line with back so fingers are pointing straight ahead and toes are pointing back. Hold a second. Return to start, then repeat with the opposite sides. That's one rep.

Push-up row (targets arms, shoulders, chest, back)

Grab a dumbbell in each hand and assume a modified push-up position with arms extended, hands under shoulders (the weights should run parallel with your body) and legs bent with your knees on the floor, ankles crossed.

Bend your elbows and lower your chest until your upper arms are parallel to the floor. Press back to start, immediately rowing the right

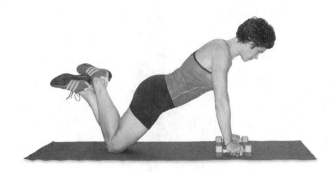

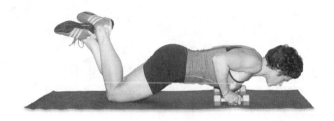

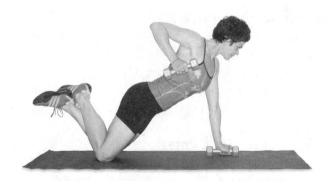

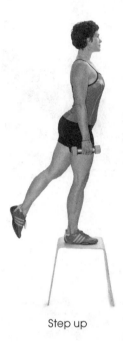

Step up

weight to your chest. Return to start and continue alternating arms for a full set.

Step up (targets legs, butt)

Stand in front of a twelve- to eighteen-inch step or bench with legs shoulder-width apart, knees slightly bent, upper body straight, and holding dumbbells down by your sides.

Step up on the step with your right foot, followed by the left foot. Step down and repeat, starting with the left foot. That's one rep.

Bridge (targets butt, core)

Lie back on the floor, knees bent and feet flat on the floor. Bring your heels as close to your butt as comfortably possible. Extend your arms down at your sides, palms flat on the floor.

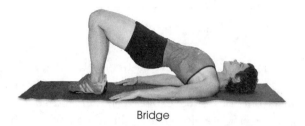

Bridge

Keeping your thighs and feet parallel, press into your feet, contract your glutes, and press your hips up toward the ceiling as far as comfortably possible.

Chair dip (targets arms, shoulders)

Sit on the edge of a sturdy chair, hands grasping the seat of the chair at either side of your rear. Walk your feet out slightly and inch your butt off the chair.

Keeping your shoulders down and your back straight, bend your elbows back and lower your butt toward the floor as far as comfortably possible. Slowly push back up.

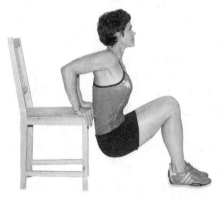

Chair dip

JUMP TO IT!

After you have four to six weeks of strength training under your belt, add some explosive "plyometric" (jumping) moves to your routine. Plyometrics build explosive power and add snap to your strength. They're also great for building bone and honing balance. Here's a move to try:

Split jump: Stand with your right leg forward and your left leg back behind you. Bend your right knee and dip your left knee toward the floor, so you're in a lunge position. Place your arms out to the sides. Swiftly jump up and switch legs. When the back knee touches the ground, jump again.

FLEXIBILITY TRAINING

Stretching is a lot like flossing. Everyone knows they should do it, but few do it as often as they should and most fib to themselves that they're going to do it more. In truth, I know plenty of cyclists who never stretch, and if it hurts their performance, you'd never know it. I also know plenty (myself included) who occasionally suffer from aches, pains, and overuse injuries that could be completely avoided with a few simple stretches.

The real deal is this: Despite all that advice from our phys. ed. teachers to stretch before working out, decades of research shows that pre-exercise stretching does nothing to prevent strains or pulls. What's more, stretching right before riding (or any athletic activity) may actually impair performance, since freshly stretched muscles produce less power and force. However, stretching does improve general flexibility and can prevent such injuries as tendonitis and iliotibial band syndrome (pain in the hips and/or knees that results from tightness in the band of tissue running between those joints), which are caused by chronic tightness. So, stretching at the end of your workout when your muscles are warm is still sound advice.

At the very least, you should take a few minutes to stretch two or three days a week the same as you do strength training. The following are six do-anywhere, cycling-specific stretches that will help keep you limber and pain free. Hold each thirty to sixty seconds.

Downward dog (targets hamstrings, calves, shoulders)

Begin on your hands and knees. Place your feet hip-width apart, with toes tucked under. Place your hands shoulder-width apart. Press your weight into your palms and straighten your legs, lifting your tailbone toward the sky while pulling your navel toward your spine and gently pushing down through the heels to stretch the back of your legs. (Keep your knees bent if this is too uncomfortable.) Keep your shoulders down and back and allow your head to hang relaxed between your arms.

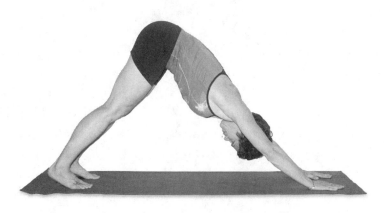

Downward dog

Figure 4 bend (targets glutes—especially the piriformis, a small muscle that runs from the base of the spine and connects to the thighbone, which gets especially tight in cyclists)

Sit in a chair with your legs bent 90 degrees and feet flat on the floor. Cross your right ankle over your left knee, so your calf is parallel to the floor and your right knee is pointing to the right. Keeping your back straight, lean forward from the hips until you feel a stretch deep in your right glute muscle. Hold, then switch legs.

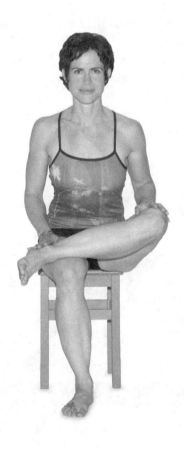

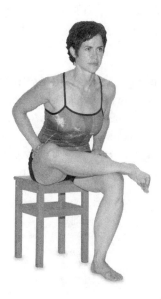

Pigeon (targets hips and quads)

Start in a kneeling position, sitting on your heels. Keeping your right knee bent, stretch your left leg back to a half-split position. (You can rest your right leg on the floor, so your right foot is positioned in front of your left hip.) Place your left knee on the floor with your leg

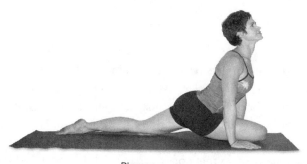

Pigeon

fully extended. Lift your head to look up at the ceiling. Place your palms down on the floor next to the right knee. Hold, then switch sides.

Butterfly (targets groin and inner thighs)

Sit on the ground with your back straight and your head up. Bend your knees to bring the soles of your feet together. Drop your knees out to the sides. Place your hands around your ankles and bend slightly forward. Using your forearms, gently press your knees toward the ground until you feel a stretch. Hold there.

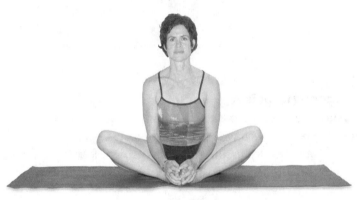

Butterfly

Cobra (targets spine and chest)

Lie facedown with your feet together, toes pointed, and your hands on the floor palms down just in front of your shoulders. Lift your chin and gently extend your arms, lifting your upper body off the floor as far as comfortably possible. If you feel any strain in your back, alter the pose so that you keep your elbows bent and forearms on the floor.

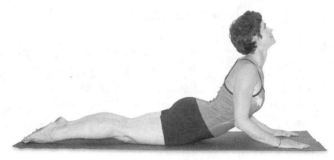

Cobra

Chest lift, shoulder squeeze (targets chest and front shoulders)

Sitting in a chair, lift your breastbone a few inches and gently squeeze your shoulder blades down and together as though you were trying to hold a pencil that is balanced along your spine.

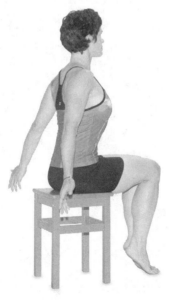

Chest lift

THE TRAINING LIFE

Once you start training, you'll likely find it hard to stop. Structure and goals are like seasoning for your riding. They spice it up and add flavor to your usual routine. Like so much in cycling, it also becomes second nature to start planning your rides and looking for progress. The great news is no matter what age you start cycling, training allows you to make great improvements and score personal bests for years to come.

7

Let's Race!

A Fun Way to Put Your Fitness to the Test

"You should race!" That's what my newfound riding friends kept telling me as we'd spin home from a spirited session. I was flattered but also dumbfounded. I wasn't a "racer." And where would I find a race even if I were interested in becoming one?

Dozens of races later, now I'm the one egging on the nimble newbies in the crowd. Not surprisingly, even all these years later, I am met with the same reaction: "Who, me?" Contrary to popular perception, racing isn't just for skinny pros without day jobs. It isn't even just for elite-level riders. It's for anyone who likes a challenge. Except for a few women at the top of the ranks, most of the women you'll be sharing the start line with are just like you. They ride for fun, and they race mostly against themselves to see how fast they can be. The only thing separating you from being a bike racer is a license. And that's just a few clicks away on the Internet.

RACING 101

There are as many different types of races as there are riders. It's important to realize that all bike races carry a measure of risk—some more than others. If you're going to race, you're going to go fast, often with many other people close by going fast too. Your chances of crashing are certainly higher than when you're riding alone. Almost every mountain bike racer I know has crashed multiple times. It's simply part of the sport. Fortunately, most crashes are minor and usually result in nothing more than a few bruises and scrapes, though broken bones can happen. Road cycling also has its share of wrecks, though I know women who race and have never wrecked.

If you're uncomfortable with riding in close quarters with other riders, are not confident in your riding ability, or are really, really afraid of falling, the majority of races are probably not for you. However, there are individual competitions you may enjoy because you aren't near other riders and can more or less race at your own comfortable pace.

Some races require that you have a license or are part of a team. Whether or not you should join a club or register yourself as a racer depends on the type of racing you'd like to do. So make that your first decision. Below are the types of races you can choose from:

ROAD RACES

As the name implies, road races are events in which people race their bikes along paved roads. If you've seen the Tour de France, you know what a (very big) road race looks like. But what you may not know is there are many other types of road race to choose from. Here's a snapshot:

Time trial

This low-risk event is the least intimidating of road races for beginners. Known as "the race against the clock" or "the race of truth" (because there's no one out there to help you; it's all you and your strength), the time trial is a race in which single riders compete on the same course to see who can complete it in the shortest length of time. Time trials can be any length; 10 miles and 40K (about 25 miles) are common distances. Riders take the course one at a time with intervals of one to two minutes separating them. You're allowed absolutely no outside help (unlike in typical road races, where teammates can give you water), and drafting (riding on the wheel of the rider in front of you, should you catch her) is not allowed. You're generally allowed to use special aero equipment, such as aerobars, that are forbidden in regular road racing.

Most time trials are individual, but there are also two-person and team time trials, where two or more riders work together to score the fastest time against similar pairs or teams.

Criterium

Criteriums, or "crits" as they're commonly called, rule the road-racing scene in the United States because they're easy to organize and require very little logistical wrangling in the way of managing traffic. A crit usually consists of a short town or city loop, generally less than 5K (about 3 miles), which is closed to traffic. You race a certain number of laps or for a certain amount of time (e.g., thirty minutes and a "bell," or final lap). Crits tend to be short—thirty to ninety minutes—so the pace is blazing. The winner is the one who crosses the finish line first without being "lapped" (passed by the lead riders). Often there are "primes" (pronounced *preeme*) or midway prizes for the winner of predetermined laps, such as every third lap.

Because they feature mass starts (meaning everyone you're racing against starts at the same time), tight corners, and high speeds, crits are very exciting and, for beginners, pretty intimidating. Good bike handling is essential. If you're interested in racing criteriums, your best bet is joining your local cycling club. Many have beginner crits where you can learn the ropes with people of like skill level.

Open road or circuit race

These are mass start races on open roads. They may run from point to point, such as one town to the next, they may follow a circuit (often ten to twenty miles in length) that you repeat, or they may be one long loop that starts and finishes at the same spot. A popular length for women's road races is about fifty miles, but they can be shorter or longer.

Though fast (after all, it is a race), road races usually run at a less intense overall pace than criteriums. You'll find people working together in groups and riding pacelines, taking turns at the front. You'll also see a lot of race tactics (see page 237) come into play. Riders will try to break away from the main group, and there's a lot of charging and chasing throughout the event. The first rider across the line wins. Open road races are somewhat less technically demanding than crits, but they still require good bike handling and awareness. Because success depends so much on group cooperation and there's a good deal of road racing etiquette to learn, joining a bike club will make your road racing experience much more enjoyable.

Stage races

Stage races are multi-day or, on the very elite level, multi-week races that typically include all the elements of racing: hilly days, flat stages, time trials, and so forth. Most stage races demand that you be part of a team. If you don't already belong to one, there may be the option of forming one online. For instance, the Tour de Toona in my home state of Pennsylvania has a Team Formation link on its Web site, so riders from all over the world can find each other and form teams. Or you could join a bike club and race as part of their team.

Track racing

I'm lucky enough to live within ten miles of a velodrome—an oval-shaped bike racing track, usually 200 to 400 meters around, made of wood or smooth cement with steep banks. Velodrome or track racing is a very special discipline done on specific bikes that have fixed gears (one speed, no coasting) and no brakes. As you might imagine, track racing demands a great deal of skill, speed, and strategy. But it's also very fun. Many tracks offer introductory programs for riders of all ages and abilities. There are only about two dozen velodromes in the United States, so they aren't easy to come by. If you ever have a chance, check it out.

WHAT TO KNOW BEFORE YOU RACE THE ROAD

If you haven't picked up on it yet, time trialing aside, road racing is very much a team sport. If you're going to join the fun, you should join a team or a club. There you'll meet other women who race with whom you can practice racing tactics and techniques such as drafting, sprinting, attacking (trying to break away and drop other riders), and peloton (group) riding. Other tips:

Buy a license

Most events allow you to purchase a single-day racing license, which is a good idea for your first time. If you're going to race more than once or twice a year, it makes economical sense to buy a license (it also helps support the sport). You can register for one through USA Cycling (www.usacycling.org), the United States' official cycling organization.

When you sign up, you'll be asked to register for a racing category. Category 1 is reserved for elite riders. Category 5 for men and Category 4 for women are the beginner categories. As you gain experience and get faster, you can work your way up the ranks. Races and events usually also divide racers by age, such as juniors for those 18 and younger, and masters and seniors for racers in older age brackets. The advantage is that racers compete against their peers, so you won't be on the line against a twenty-two-year-old college stud who has nothing but time to train.

Know the rules

Confession: I competed in my first road race in a baggy T-shirt that I'd cut down to size with a pocketknife. It wasn't a bad fashion statement left over from the '80s; it was because I came to the race wearing a tank top—an official no-no. Race rules state that all participants' shoulders must be covered. Having only raced mountain bike events (where riders wear everything but their birthday suits . . . and sometimes even that), I had no clue. A very friendly race official pulled out his Swiss Army knife, and we fashioned a makeshift jersey out of one of the event tees. It was lovely. You'll get a rulebook along with your license. It's a good idea to read it.

Get in the loop

New racers always want to know how to find races. Bike clubs are one way. Another way is the Internet. Sites such as www.active.com are hotbeds of information on events and races around the country. Just pick your sport and plug in your zip code, and you'll find a surprising array of cycling events happening in your area. You can also sign up to receive online announcements of events going on near you.

OFF-ROAD RACES

As you might guess, off-road races are just that, bike races that take place off of paved surfaces, usually on mountain bikes (though there are some exceptions). The terrain varies widely from fire roads to dirt paths to rocky, root-filled trails deep in the woods. Because of the rugged terrain and burly bikes, the speed in mountain biking racing is often half that of a road race, but the effort is certainly no less intense. Like road racing, there are many different types of off-road event to choose from. Here are the main selections:

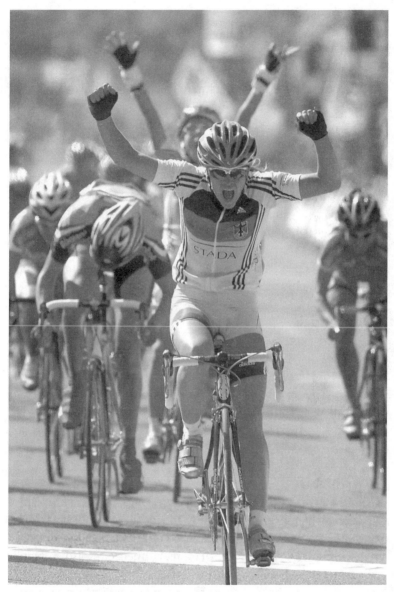

Germany's Regina Schleicher, cyclist for Fuji, celebrates her win at the 2005 World Road Cycling Championships in Madrid, Spain.

Cross-country

Cross-country ("XC") mountain bike races are generally off-road circuit races, where riders race around a loop anywhere from three to ten miles long. How many times you go around the loop depends on your race experience; beginners may just do one or two laps, while experts go around five or six times. Most cross-country courses aren't terribly technical, but they may definitely include some challenging sections with rocks, roots, logs, and/or steep descents.

Most cross-country races last about two hours, and they start very fast. After the start, the pack generally thins out, and you spend most of the race out there with a small group of riders. Some mountain bikers have teams, but it's much more of an individual sport than road cycling. Mountain bikers for the most part are not allowed outside assistance (although that has changed on the professional level, and some races make exceptions), and you rarely see mountain bikers working together tactically the way road cyclists do.

Short track

Short-track cross-country mountain bike races are basically off-road criteriums. The courses tend to be very short, so they're good for spectators (you can often see much of the race while standing in one spot). They're often run by time, so instead of doing a certain number of laps, you race for thirty minutes plus a "bell" (final) lap. The winner is the rider who crosses the line first with the most laps completed.

Marathon

As the name implies, these events are *long,* some even as long as 100 miles (which is a *very long* way to ride a mountain bike). Fifty-milers are also popular. These arduous events usually last for the better part of a day. Though less common, there are also mountain biking stage racing events, where riders travel from point A to point B over a specified number of days. These multi-day races have a reputation as being the toughest competitions the sport has to offer.

24-hour and Enduro

Off-road 24-hour races are some of the most popular mountain biking events. Though some people do them solo, most often it is a team competition. Teams can consist of two, four, or sometimes five riders, most often a group of friends who come together just for the race and come up with a funny team name like 4 Fat Guys Who Like Beer. Team members take turns riding laps around a racecourse over a twenty-four-hour period (usually noon on a Saturday until noon the next Sunday). Yes, that means you ride through the night with lights on your helmet and bike. These races are usually held at ski resorts or other camp-friendly venues and are known for their very laid-back festival atmosphere as racers camp out and cheer each other on.

Enduros are similar in spirit but aren't necessarily twenty-four hours in length. Many are six or twelve hours in length, which makes them great for people who like competing in long events but don't necessarily want to camp out or ride at night. Some are team events; others are for solo riders only.

Downhill

Downhill mountain biking is so radically different from XC racing that it's practically a different sport. The bikes are much bigger and heavier, and riders wear full-face helmets and light body armor that includes knee and shin pads, shoulder pads, and sometimes even spine protection. Downhill racing is a time trial–style event, where riders take a ski lift (with their bikes) to the top of a mountain and take turns seeing who can get down a designated trail in the fastest time. Races last anywhere from less than a minute to about six minutes, depending on the course and the competition level. The courses are highly technical and include steep drop-offs and tight turns through rocks and trees.

Other forms of downhill racing include dual slalom (two riders competing side by side), four cross (four riders competing on the same course to the finish), and Super D (aka Super Downhill), a mix of cross-country and downhill. Downhill racing tends to be male dominated, but women do compete, and some of the most accomplished women in mountain biking have raced in this discipline.

Cyclocross

Developed as an off-season training tool for European road racers, 'cross races could be considered an off-road race for roadies. The courses are unpaved, but most competitors compete on road bikes (or special cyclocross bikes, which are a beefy type of road bike; see page 17), though mountain bikes are allowed. Cyclocross is done on a short loop that racers compete around for 40 to 45 minutes plus a "bell" (final) lap. Courses include man-made barriers like hurdles and stairs that force competitors to dismount and run with their bikes for short stretches to clear the obstacles before remounting. Races are held in the fall, and mud, rain, and even snow are common.

WHAT TO KNOW BEFORE YOU RACE OFF-ROAD

Though there are certainly some very serious mountain bike competitors, mountain bike races on the whole have a much more laid-back atmosphere than road races. Because most racers compete as individuals rather than on teams, you find a wider array of athletes and abilities; most are there just to have a good time. If you're intimidated by the thought of going it alone, find a club that has a mountain bike division or, better yet, a specific mountain bike club. Ask your bike shop about ones in your area. Other things to know:

License?

If you're going to participate in NORBA (National Off-Road Bicycling Association) races, which fall under the USA Cycling umbrella, you need a USA Cycling–issued license to compete. You can usually purchase single-day licenses on a race-by-race basis, but, as with road racing, if you're doing a whole series of events, it's best to support the sport and buy a license. Unlike road racing, however, where nearly every race requires a license, mountain biking is rife with unofficial races put on by independent race organizers where no license is required. License requirements will be clear on the race application.

Find your event

Mountain bike races can be a little trickier to find, since they often don't show up on mainstream event-finders like www.active.com. Better places to check are sport-specific sites, including www.mountainbike racer.com, which focus on off-road events around the country. Your bike shop or local bike club also can help you find events.

RACE PREPARATION AND TACTICAL SMARTS

It's natural to feel like you've swallowed a bucketful of dragonflies the morning before a race. Races are high-stress situations (even if you're not really *competing*, you'll get swept up in the excitement), which bring out the best, and sometimes worst, in people. Your goal is to keep your head on straight, come ready to compete, and race fair and square. Many of the finer nuances of racing are best learned on the bike with other riders. So I'll say it again: If you're serious about racing, particularly road racing, join a club. In the meantime, here are a few tips that will help:

MAKE A LIST AND CHECK IT TWICE

The night before your race (or earlier if you can), make a list of what you need (see below), double-check it, and pack up. You don't want to be running around like a madwoman searching for your socks the morning of the event. Also do a quick bike check. Check that the tires are inflated and the bike is shifting smoothly. Do not make any major adjustments, perform any intense cleaning, or put anything new on the bike. You want to race your bike as you've been training on it.

Pack thoroughly

What should you bring? Everything, within reason. To be well prepared, include:

- Helmet (can't race without one)
- Jersey and shorts (or, if you're going to wear them there, put them out). If there are any dress codes (such as no sleeveless jerseys), know about them in advance.
- Cycling shoes and socks
- Gloves
- Glasses
- Water bottles (for road race) or hydration backpack (for mountain race)
- Food, water, sports drink (whatever you plan on eating/drinking before, during, and after the event). Do not pack any unfamiliar foods or drink. Only use what you've trained on and know that your body tolerates well under high-intensity efforts.
- Tools. At minimum you should have a spare tube, pump, and tire levers.
- Wallet with necessary money, ID, and license, if necessary. (Inevitably, people show up without these; I've done it. It stinks.)
- Paperwork. Bring your directions to the venue, along with any important paperwork the race director may have sent in advance (e.g., confirmation numbers).

ARRIVE EARLY, WARM UP THOROUGHLY

Plan to get to the race venue at least an hour and a half early; earlier is even better, especially if this is your first race. There's a lot to negotiate at race venues, including parking, sign-in or registration, race packet pickup, fastening race numbers to your bike and/or jersey, potty stops, and so on. Leave yourself plenty of time so you don't feel rushed.

Once you're signed in and set up, go out and ride around the venue. Or, if you're at a mountain bike event or a criterium, pre-ride the course—yes, take a full lap around the course (provided, of course, it's only a few miles long and there's not an earlier race in progress). Your warm-up intensity should be easy to moderate with a few short hard efforts to get your legs going. Way too many new racers miss out on the advantages of a proper warm-up because they don't want to "wear themselves out" for the race. A good warm-up burns off the pre-race jitters, warms your muscles, fires up your fat-burning enzymes, and calms your mind. Skip this step and your body is forced to use the first fifteen or twenty minutes of the race to get in gear.

PACE YOURSELF . . . TO A POINT

Race pacing is an art. Even well-seasoned competitors sometimes charge out too hard and blow up before the finish, or finish with too much energy to spare and feel like they missed out by not going hard enough. Use your head. If it's only ten minutes into the race and you feel terrible, back off, breathe deep, and regain your composure. If you're feeling great, push it, but try to avoid going too far into the red (where you're heavily gasping for breath) too often too early. A hard push to make it up a particularly challenging climb is fine, but you can't stay at max intensity for too long and expect to finish strong. Your pace should feel hard but not impossibly so.

Most coaches will advise you not to start too hard. That's good advice. But in mountain bike races, it could cost you a win if you're gunning for first place. Many mountain bike courses start on an open field and then follow a road (often up a hill) for a quarter mile or so before diving into the woods, where the course narrows and passing becomes difficult, if not impossible. In these situations, the racers gun it from the line as hard as humanly possible to get the coveted "hole shot" (first racer into the woods). You don't need the hole shot to win, but it sure does help you get a firm advantage on the field.

RACE WITH GRACE

The vast majority of racers and volunteers are just like you: men and women with day jobs who are pursuing an activity they love. Respect them, including those you are competing against. People do dumb things in the heat of competition. You may get cut off by a rider ahead of you or another rider may be in your way fixing a flat on the trail. It's okay to firmly address the situation by yelling "Rider coming through!" if you want someone to move off the path, or "Slowing!" if you need to slam on the brakes during a road race. But don't swear, berate, or be confrontational. And if someone is rude to you, shrug it off as the act of someone who doesn't know how to behave with grace under pressure. When possible, shout some thanks to the volunteers. Without them, you wouldn't be there.

LAUNCHING AND COVERING AN ATTACK

Road racing is all about tactics. One of the most common techniques—and one you'll want to know going in—is the attack. Small groups will accelerate to try to break away from the main field; others usually then chase after them to reel them back in. Though some individuals attack on their lonesome for no apparent reason, most often attacks are strategically planned to help a rider or group of riders get away from the pack and have fewer competitors with whom they need to contend for the finish line at the end.

Before you attack, consider what you hope to gain. Is the race winding down and you feel like you can stay away until the end? Are you a stellar climber and feel confident you can beat everyone up a tough climb and gain time on your competitors? Are you trying to wear out the competition so a teammate can steal the lead down the road? Don't waste energy attacking just because you feel you should. Have a purpose in mind.

Time your attacks wisely. It doesn't make much sense to launch an attack when you know that thirty people will be on your wheel within seven seconds. Plan your attacks at hard points in the race, such as the top of a tough climb when many riders are giving their all and won't have energy to try to chase you down. Realize of course there will be plenty of times when you'll be the one watching someone ride off into the distance because they attacked when you had no energy to spare. That's just the nature of the game.

Finally, know when to say when. If you attack and a few riders follow, that's good. You'll have a small group to share the work as you try to maintain your breakaway. If you're struggling to stay off the front of the field and a mass of humanity is closing in on you, don't waste your energy fighting the inevitable. Sit up and rejoin the fold.

What if you're on the other side of the attack? You have to decide if you consider them a real threat (i.e., will they be able to maintain their lead to the end?) and if you have the energy to chase them down and match their speed. Like so many of the finer points of riding and racing, this is one that you'll learn through trial and error and, even then, still won't always get it just right. That's the fun and spirit of the sport.

Mountain bike races tend to spread out, and you rarely find yourself in a pack. But you will likely find yourself dueling with a few other racers throughout the event. The attacking tactics are similar. Try to drop them when you feel they're most weak, such as hard climbs or rocky, technical sections. With mountain bike racing in particular, you can be at a great advantage if you can break away just far enough that the competitor behind you can't see you and doesn't have you in her sights to chase. But don't waste too much energy when you are evenly matched. Save yourself for a big push at the end.

SHARE THE WORK

When you're in a group, even in a race, riders will often take turns pulling at the front, then drifting back to take a break and draft with the pack. But there are no hard and fast rules here. Sometimes teams will take the front and try to dominate. Sometimes they'll try to force other riders to the front in order to save their energies. You can discuss strategy with your teammates ahead of time.

If you're part of a breakaway group, however, you'll find that the group generally does more sharing of the work to keep the speed higher and maintain distance from the pack. But, again, if you're alone with no teammates among other racers and their teammates, you're at a distinct disadvantage, and you shouldn't expect a whole lot of help out there.

PASS WITH CARE

Passing riders on a wide, closed road is easy, so there's generally no reason to announce your intentions (in fact, it's best to use the element of surprise). Just remember to keep your movements steady. You don't want to swerve all over the road or cut other riders off. Off-road, where riders are skirting around rocks and roots and can't be expected to ride a perfectly straight line, it's another story. Announce "On your left" or "On your right" to let riders know you'll be coming by and what side to expect you on.

SIT IN AND ENJOY THE SHOW

Maybe it's just not your day, or maybe it's never really your day. You can still "compete and complete," which is what most midpack riders do at most events. You show up, ride your best, and finish somewhere in the field, maybe even last (hey, someone has to be the caboose). Every rider who crosses a finish line should feel proud for having the guts to have even started.

HOW'D IT GO OUT THERE?

Hindsight, as they say, is always 20/20. After a race, it's easy to sit back and evaluate what went right or wrong. Then it's back to training to work on what you need to do better the next time.

If you start to get serious, you can also consider hiring a coach. There are many online coaching services that will provide you with a coach who will help you assess your skills, build a training plan, and dramatically improve your race results.

You can also keep it casual and just go out to see what you can do without worrying about final results. Racing is a fun way to give more meaning to your everyday rides. Winning medals or coming across the finish line with your fastest time ever are enormously satisfying, but, in the end, racing should be a means to itself—a way to challenge yourself, have a good time, and become a better bicyclist in the process.

8

Cycling Food

Fuel Up to Ride Strong and Feel Great

There's a saying in cycling circles: We eat to ride and ride to eat. Two hours of brisk recreational riding (at about 12 MPH) burns about 1,000 calories—half a day's worth! So it's little wonder that cyclists enjoy plenty of food both on and off the bike.

As elementary as the act of eating is, the biggest mistakes new (and many not so new) cyclists make center around food. Namely, they don't eat enough of the right foods at the right times. Your bike might have lots of fancy gears and components, but you are the engine that makes it go, and that engine needs the right mix of fuel to keep running strong.

ESSENTIAL EATS FOR ENERGY AND REPAIR

On a very basic level, food serves two purposes for your cycling body: It provides energy for your working muscles while you're riding, and it helps restock your fuel stores and repair your muscles when you're done. The three main fuel sources you get from food are carbohydrates, protein, and fat. Here's how they work:

CARBOHYDRATES GET (AND KEEP) YOU GOING

The low-carb mania of recent years was blown monumentally out of proportion (swearing off apples and carrots? Please!), but it *did* serve some benefit: It taught us that all carbs are not created equal and that contrary to the low-fat, high-carb hysteria of the '90s, carbs alone will not answer your weight loss prayers. As a cyclist, you'll be consuming plenty of the right kinds of carbs . . . and staying slim.

Carbohydrates, which are found in abundance in grain-based foods like cereal, pasta, breads, and baked goods as well as fruits and vegetables and even dairy foods like milk, are your body's best fuel. After you eat them, your body quickly breaks them down into blood sugar called glucose. Your hungry cells suck up this blood sugar and convert it into energy. What you don't use immediately goes into short-term storage as muscle glycogen or gets converted to fat to burn down the road.

Your body burns carbohydrates at every exercise intensity. About 50 to 60% of your energy comes from stored carbs during easy riding, and nearly all your energy comes from this quick-burning fuel during vigorous efforts. Most of us store about 1,800 calories' worth of carbs in our muscles, blood, and liver. A fast ride can burn more than 600 calories an hour, and you don't want to deplete those stores to zero, so it's important to keep the carbs coming in a steady supply. If you're planning to ride longer than 90 minutes, the point at which your muscle glycogen stores start resembling bakery bins before a blizzard, you should bring some food or carb-containing sports drink with you to top off your tank.

Carbohydrates come in two forms. The first is simple carbs, like fruit (fructose), milk (lactose), honey (fructose and glucose), and table sugar (sucrose), which are composed of just one or two sugar molecules.

The second is complex carbs, like whole grains, starches (e.g., potatoes), beans, and other plant foods, which are made up of long chains of sugar molecules. But, contrary to popular belief, simple carbs aren't necessarily any more "fast-acting" than complex carbs, nor are they more "fattening" (another myth). What really matters when you're weighing the value of your carbohydrate is the other nutrients found in the food and how much processing it's been through.

Unprocessed carbs like fruits and whole-grain cereals that are rich in fiber and nutrients not only supply your active body with the vitamins and minerals it needs to stay healthy; they also tend to digest more slowly and provide even energy (blood sugar) levels. Highly refined carbs like cakes and chips and white-flour baked goods, on the other hand, send your blood sugar soaring, triggering an insulin spike that pulls so much glucose (sugar) out of your bloodstream you end up feeling hungry again soon after. There *is* a time and a place for these superfast sugar sources, but keep them to a minimum in your daily diet.

The simplest rule for eating smart carbs is to eat as close to nature as possible. The more recognizable and less processed a food is, the better. Whole fruits, vegetables, and grains are always a winner. Look for pastas, breads, and other baked goods that contain whole grains, not refined flour.

The average cyclist needs about 400 to 450 grams of carbs a day. That may sound like a truckload, but when you consider that one cup of fruit yogurt delivers 50 grams, it adds up fast. While you're at it, aim for 25 to 35 grams of fiber (abundant in smart carb sources). Fiber increases the satiety in food (meaning you feel full longer) and reduces the number of calories your body absorbs, so it's excellent for shedding excess pounds. Most Americans eat only about 13 grams a day, far less than they need. Here are some examples of excellent sources:

CARBOHYDRATES		
Food	Carbs	Fiber
Baked potato with skin (1 medium)	60 grams	6.6 grams
Oatmeal (1 cup)	25 grams	4 grams
Lentil soup (1 cup)	20 grams	5.6 grams
Raisin bran (1 cup)	42 grams	5 grams
Whole wheat pasta (1 cup)	37 grams	6.3 grams
Apple (1 large)	29 grams	5 grams

PROTEIN FOR REPAIR

Protein is composed of twenty different amino acids, which in turn act as the building blocks for your muscles. This essential macronutrient also helps build immunity and repairs and maintains all types of bodily tissue. The body can't store protein as it can carbs and fat, so it's essential to eat enough every day, especially as you start riding more.

Though cyclists often don't place as heavy a premium on protein as their peers in power-based sports, endurance athletes need every bit as much of this muscle maker. On long rides your brain and muscles use protein as supplemental fuel (especially when you're running low on carbs). About 5% of your energy needs are supplied by amino acids, specifically leucine, isoleucine, and valine. Your muscles also need a constant supply of protein for repair. Endurance athletes like cyclists should eat a minimum of 0.5 grams of protein for every pound of body weight, or about 70 grams for a 140-pound woman. The average American woman comes in a little shy of that at about 63 grams a day.

Like carbs, proteins come in two forms: complete and incomplete. As the name implies, complete proteins contain all the essential amino acids your body needs to make muscle and per-form other functions. All animal products are complete proteins. Soybeans are also a complete protein source. Incomplete proteins are usually heavy in some amino acids but completely lacking in others, so they need to be combined with other incomplete pro-teins to form a whole protein source. Plant foods such as beans, grains, seeds, and nuts tend to be incomplete proteins. But as long as you eat a wide variety of incomplete proteins, such as beans and rice and even peanut butter and bread, within the same day, your body will get what it needs.

Though everyone agrees that active people need plenty of protein, there's tremendous debate in the sports nutrition field as to how much protein you need *during* exercise. Some researchers have found that a small amount of protein taken during exercise (usually in the form of a sports drink) helps reduce muscle damage and increases endurance. But others have failed to find a benefit. On long bike tours (for example, a 500-mile ride my husband and I did across part of Montana), I find a carb-protein energy drink can keep my legs feeling fresher from day to day.

The most important amino acids for endurance exercisers appear to be leucine, isoleucine, and valine, since they're the ones that your muscles oxidize to make energy. In one study published in the *European Journal of Applied Physiology,* researchers found that canoeists who popped leucine for six weeks improved the time they could row until exhaustion by *eleven minutes.* Even better: They reported a lower rating of perceived exertion while doing it. They rowed longer but felt like the work was easier. You can't beat that.

Though protein isn't the weight loss miracle high-protein propo-nents paint it to be, it does seem to help whittle your waistline. A study published in *The Journal of Nutrition* reported that exercisers who were trying to lose weight were able to maintain lean muscle tis-sue and lose fat faster when they emphasized such high-quality pro-tein food as eggs, lean meats, and low-fat dairy and avoided high-carb fare including pasta, potatoes, and bread.

Finally, research suggests that various amino acids may boost immunity, protect against overtraining, keep legs fresher during exercise and help them recover faster, elevate mood, and sharpen mental function during endurance activities like century bike rides.

The easiest way to get the amino acids your active body needs is to eat some protein with every meal. Here are some outstanding sources:

PROTEINS	
Food	**Protein**
Eggs (2)	12 grams
Low-fat milk (1 cup)	8 grams
Cheese (2 oz.)	14 grams
Tuna (6 oz.)	40 grams
Chicken breast (3 oz.)	24 grams
Pork chop (3 oz.)	24 grams
Lean beef (3 oz., cooked)	21 grams
Tofu, firm (1/2 block)	26 grams
Salmon (3 oz.)	19 grams
Lentils (1 cup, cooked)	18 grams
Soy milk (1 cup)	11 grams
Peanut butter (2 Tbsp.)	8 grams

FAT FOR THE LONG HAUL

Like carbs, fat was widely demonized as a waistline wrecker before folks came to understand that not all fat is bad, and just because you eat fat doesn't mean you'll get fat. Unfortunately, this message hasn't fully sunken in for many endurance athletes (like cyclists), who still banish this essential substance and suffer unintended consequences.

First, it's important to recognize that muscles do not run on carbs alone. Your muscles store fat just as they store carbs, which they use as fuel for light to moderate intensity exercise. The right mix of carbs, fat, and protein feeds your muscles as you pedal at varying intensities and helps stretch out your glycogen stores so they last longer while you're out on the road. That's especially true as you become more fit. The better shape you're in, the better your body becomes at burning fat, even at higher intensities, so you can ride longer and harder without "bonking" (running out of energy from poor fueling).

Fact is, it's hard to beat fat as a fuel source. Fat packs more than twice the energy per gram as either carbs or protein (that's where the low-fat diet craze came from). Just one pound of stored fat contains enough energy to fuel a six-hour ride (if you burned 100% fat, which, of course, you don't). Most of us stockpile in the neighborhood of 60,000 calories' worth of this slow-burning energy source, because historically we had to survive famines. Fat is an outstanding energy source and not one for cyclists to be particularly stingy about including on their plates. Studies show endurance exercisers perform significantly better on a diet that has about 30% of its calories from fat than a lower 20% one.

Fat in your diet also helps you absorb essential antioxidants including vitamins A, D, E, and K, and beta-carotene. Your body depends on fat to produce hormones like estrogen and testosterone and to build nerve tissue. What's important is that you eat the right amount of the right kinds of fat.

There are good fats, great fats, okay fats, and downright terrible fats. Some clog up your arteries, while others help keep them healthy and clean. Some appear to fire up your metabolism, while others may slow it down. A few are good for some things and bad for others. Following is a guide to cut through the confusion.

Unsaturated fats

The best of the best, these are the fats found in plant foods and fish. They come in two forms:

- **Monounsaturated:** Abundant in olive, canola, and peanut oil as well as nuts and avocados, these super healthy fats lower low-density lipoprotein cholesterol (LDL, or "bad cholesterol") while raising or maintaining healthful high-density lipoprotein cholesterol (HDL, or "good cholesterol").

- **Polyunsaturated:** These are mostly healthy, though some types of polyunsaturated fats can slightly lower HDL cholesterol when eaten in high amounts. The poly fats include the essential fatty acids omega-3 and omega-6. As you've likely heard, omega-3 fatty acids protect against a host of illnesses including heart disease, autoimmune diseases, certain cancers, arthritis, and maybe Alzheimer's disease. Some animal research also suggests that omega-3s actually promote fat metabolism and discourage unhealthy fat storage. Yet most of us don't eat enough of them because they're found in fish and flaxseed, neither of which is a staple in most Americans' diets. Omega-6 fatty acids are abundant in seeds and vegetable oils. Most Americans eat way more omega-6 fatty acids than they need in the form of fried food.

Saturated fats

These fats found mainly in animal fats (meats, full-fat dairy foods, butter, etc.) have traditionally been bundled in the "bad fat" category. But new research shows that though they tend to be less healthy as a whole, they're anything but all bad. Coconut oil, which is a saturated fat, seems to act more like unsaturated fat in your body. And some saturated fatty acids may actually improve your cholesterol profile. So while it's best to keep saturated fats in check, there's no need to eliminate them entirely.

Trans fats

With entire cities passing legislation to ban them, you know they're bad. Trans fats occur in very small amounts in nature (natural sources seem to be okay), but more often than not they come in the form of hydrogenated (solidified) or partially hydrogenated vegetable oils, which are awful for you. They've not only been found to cause hardening of the arteries and heart disease, but a growing body of research suggests that they promote weight gain and encourage the body to store dangerous abdominal fat even if you're not eating more calories. Until very recently, they were abundant in processed, packaged, and fried foods like crackers, cookies, cake frosting, and chips as well as shortening and margarine. Today manufacturers are making a concerted effort to eliminate them.

But buyer beware. You'll see plenty of packages trumpeting "Trans Fat Free!" in the grocery stores, but even snack foods that claim to be trans fat can contain up to a half a gram per serving. It doesn't take long for that to add up if you eat lots of these foods. If the ingredients include partially hydrogenated vegetable oil, hydrogenated vegetable oil, or vegetable shortening, the food contains trans fat.

For optimal performance, aim to eat about 30% of your calories from healthy fats. If you eat 2,000 calories a day, that's about 65 grams preferably in the form of plant foods, fish, healthy oils, lean meats and poultry, and low-fat dairy foods. Here are some good sources:

GOOD FATS	
Food	**Fat**
Eggs (2 scrambled)	15 grams
Mixed nuts (1 oz.)	14.5 grams
Salmon (3 oz.)	10.5 grams
Tofu (½ block)	14 grams
Peanut butter (2 Tbsp.)	16 grams
Olive oil (1 Tbsp.)	13.5 grams
Avocado (½ a fruit)	14 grams

DRINK UP!

The average 140-pound woman can easily shed 2 pounds of water during a hot summer ride. Easy weight loss, right? Wrong. Dehydration slows you down, so you perform poorly and burn fewer calories.

When you sweat a lot without replenishing your fluids, your blood volume decreases, which makes your heart work harder. Experts estimate that for every pound of sweat you lose, your heart rate increases about eight beats per minute. Your body's ability to cool itself also diminishes, so your core body temperature inches up. Sweat out two pounds or more and even a ride to the beach feels like a march across Bataan.

Most bikes come with attachments for two bottles. Use them. As a rule of thumb, you should be drinking at least 3 or 4 ounces every 15 minutes (more if it's very hot or you're out for a long day, such as for a century ride); that's a 12- to 16-ounce water bottle an hour. Drinking at this rate may not completely replace every ounce of fluid you lose. That's okay. Your goal is simply to stay ahead of dehydration, not drown yourself. In recent years some recreational athletes have taken the message to stay hydrated way too far and have made themselves sick (in a few cases fatally so) with too much water.

Speaking of water, plain fluid's okay for short easy rides. But for anything longer than that, or even hour-long outings in very hot and humid conditions, take a sports drink. Every pound of sweat contains precious electrolyte minerals, specifically sodium, potassium, magnesium, and calcium, which work together to fire your muscles, regulate nerve transmission, and maintain the body's delicate fluid balance. Sweat out enough and you suffer the consequences of fatigue, cramping, and nausea. Sports drinks are specially formulated to replace electrolytes (as well as carbohydrates). They also hydrate you better than water because the added sodium encourages your body to retain water (instead of peeing it out) and encourages you to drink more.

Which sports drink should you choose? Honestly, they all work. Studies show any carbohydrate beverage improves performance. So, it comes down to personal preference. Just don't make the mistake of substituting iced tea, juice, soda, or another everyday beverage for your specially formulated sports drink. Many soft drinks and juices easily contain twice as much sugar (carbs) as a sports drink like Gatorade. All that sugar slows digestion and water absorption and can leave you with a sloshing, queasy stomach.

TIMING IS EVERYTHING

I'll never forget my first century. Not only for the rolling, misty roads dotted with horses and buggies carrying dozens of Mennonites to an early morning wedding but because it was the first time I ever "bonked."

Bonking is the term cyclists use for hitting the wall. It happens when your liver glycogen stores run dry and you have no more fuel to feed your brain, which, like your muscles, runs on stored carbs. It's a feeling of profound fatigue and utter despair. And it comes seemingly out of nowhere.

Though I had plowed through piles of spaghetti the night before and eaten an ample stack of pancakes before we rolled out, I didn't eat anything more than a few pretzel sticks and some Gatorade for the first fifty miles. When we got to the lunch stop, we were greeted with stale bagels and peanut butter and jelly. The lunch truck carrying our subs and snacks had broken down. I shrugged it off. Still so excited by the sights and experience, I wasn't all that hungry anyway, so I halfheartedly snacked on a few bites of bagel and rolled off. I was fine . . . until mile 75. Suddenly I felt like I couldn't pedal another stroke. I asked my husband how much farther we had to go. "I think ten miles," he said, trying to encourage me. I burst into tears. Someone gave me part of an energy bar, but it wasn't enough. I spent the remainder of the ride pitifully weeping and feeling like the worst cyclist ever.

When we finally pulled into the finish line feed stations, I inhaled six slices of pizza and vowed never to bonk again. The take-home message is it's not just what you eat but *when*. The following is a guide for fueling before, during, and after the ride. (Note: These rules really only apply to rides of longer durations or short, intense efforts like a race. If you're going out for an hour or two of easy spinning or less than ninety minutes of more moderate to intense riding, you should be fine eating and snacking as you normally do.)

BEFORE YOU RIDE: CARBO-LOADING AND BEYOND

When you're gearing up for a big ride—a century, triathlon, or mountain bike adventure—you need to start stocking your stores well before the event. Too many riders mistakenly treat the food they eat the morning of a ride or race as their fuel for the day, when the fuel your body uses is glycogen that is neatly tucked away in your muscles from meals eaten as long as eight to twelve hours prior.

The concept of carbo-loading has come to mean stuffing your stomach with as many dinner rolls and ziti servings as it will hold the night before a big event. What you really should be doing is not necessarily eating more, but about two days out from the event, start skewing your meals to focus more, but heavily on carbohydrates. The real key here is tapering your activity so the carbs that you'd usually burn off by riding are used to fill your glycogen stores to full capacity. Studies show this tapering-glycogen loading strategy can improve performance by 2 to 3%. More important, it makes you feel rested, energized, and ready to go.

The morning of your event (preferably about two and half to three hours before), eat a high-carb, easy-to-digest breakfast of about 400 to 500 calories. If your event is really early, don't wake up at four a.m. just to eat. Just be sure you've eaten a healthy, carb-heavy dinner and eat a smaller breakfast, say a 200-calorie energy bar, an hour or so before your early morning event. But whatever you do, don't skip breakfast. A morning meal is essential for topping off your liver glycogen stores, which get used up quickly overnight and will be at least half empty come morning even if you feasted at Pasta Palace the night before. A bowl of oatmeal, a cup of cold cereal, or two pancakes with a piece of fruit and half a cup of yogurt will also give your blood sugar (and energy levels) a quick boost, stave off hunger, and improve performance. In one study, a group of cyclists who ate carbs before riding were able to pedal 18% longer before fatiguing.

DURING THE RIDE

For rides longer than 90 minutes, bring some carbs along in the form of sports drink, energy bars, or energy gels. Sports nutritionists recommend eating about 100 to 300 calories (depending on the intensity of your efforts) of carbohydrates per hour of riding after the first 60 to 90 minutes. Energy gels like GU and ClifShot and bars like PowerBar and LUNA make keeping up with your carb needs a snap. One gel (a small packet of flavored syrup) or half a bar typically contains about 100 calories of carbs. Wash it down with some energy drink, which delivers about 50 calories per 8 ounces, and you're good to keep going. Remember, your brain needs fuel too. Researchers have found that exercisers who keep their blood sugar levels up with a sports drink feel happier and more energized than those who try to get by on plain water alone.

POST-RIDE

Rides lasting more than 90 minutes deplete your glycogen stores (as do very hard rides of shorter duration), which your muscles need for post-exercise recovery and repair. You can increase the rate of muscle repair three-fold and triple the rate at which your muscles restock their stores by eating a blend of carbohydrates and protein within 30 minutes of a hard ride, when your body is still revved up and is in high-speed refueling and repair mode.

Since the goal is to pour glucose into your hungry cells, now is a fine time to indulge in your favorite fast-digesting refined carbs. Some good post-ride snacks include a bagel and peanut butter, a plate of spaghetti, or maybe best of all chocolate milk (I'm a huge

Ovaltine fan, since it's also fortified with vitamins and minerals and makes a guilt-free mocha). For years racers have sworn by finishing a hard day with this sweet drink. Now research shows chocolate milk works just as well as, if not better than, pricey specially formulated recovery drinks. One study found that cyclists who drank low-fat chocolate milk after an exhausting ride were able to pedal about 50% longer during a second ride four hours later than those who drank other beverages.

Another great recovery option is a smoothie. The right ice-cold blend delivers a healing combination of carbs, protein, and antioxidant-filled fruit, while also helping you rehydrate post ride. Here's a simple recipe:

Cycling Smoothie

Mix the following ingredients in a blender until smooth. Experiment by adding vanilla, cinnamon, nutmeg, or other flavorings:

> 1 cup skim milk
> 1/2 frozen banana
> 1 tsp. honey
> 1 cup your favorite frozen fruit (try strawberries, pineapple chunks, or blueberries)

AVOID TUMMY TROUBLES

Unlike runners, who literally jostle their stomach up and down with every step, cyclists can get away with eating almost anything very close to and during their activity. The key word is *almost*. If your ride includes a lot of high-intensity efforts like intervals or hills, you may need to be more careful. I learned the hard way (twice) that I don't tolerate bananas (a cyclist staple) before high-intensity rides. Other riders swear off eggs. Unfortunately, sports nutrition is always a bit of trial and error. But there are some guidelines that can help.

As a rule, anything you eat before a strenuous ride, when your blood is going to be too busy delivering oxygen to your legs to help out with digestion, should be light and bland. Fatty foods (like cream-filled donuts) will sit like a lump in your stomach during high-intensity efforts. Protein also slows digestion, so a protein bar or a club sandwich isn't your best choice either. Pancakes, cereal, energy bars, bagels, and fig bars are some safe staples. Also avoid acidic foods like oranges, which can disrupt digestion and leave you feeling queasy when you ride.

PERFORMANCE ENHANCERS

Elite-level cyclists are known to pop all sorts of supplements from simple protein powders to dried Asian mushrooms and other mysterious herbs to improve performance. There's some evidence that supports the use of certain ergogenic (supposedly performance enhancing) aids, but, truthfully, there's very little hard science on many of these substances.

What we do know is that micronutrients like vitamins and minerals and other everyday food components can keep your muscles healthy and your energy high. We also know that active women often run low on some of the essentials. Here's what to watch for:

VITAMINS AND MINERALS

All the carbs, protein, and healthy fat in the world will do you little good without the proper amounts of vitamins and minerals to metabolize them. Recent research shows that athletes (yes, that includes recreational cyclists) don't perform their best and may have trouble building muscle and producing oxygen-carrying red blood cells if they're low in B vitamins (e.g., B6, B12, folate, and riboflavin), which are essential for converting protein and sugar to energy and for repairing cells.

Unfortunately, women are at risk for dipping dangerously close to deficiency in a number of essential vitamins and minerals because they often skimp on such nutrient-dense foods like nuts, breads, and dairy in hopes of shedding weight. Though popping a daily multivitamin is good insurance, the only way to feed your body what it needs is through fresh, whole foods, which contain not only all the essential nutrients but also dozens of other protective antioxidants scientists are only beginning to understand. As an active woman, you should aim for *at least* five servings of fruits and vegetables a day.

Active women also need to be particularly vigilant about calcium and iron—essential minerals for building bone and blood. The average adult gets only about 700 milligrams of calcium a day, way short of the recommended amount of 1,000 to 1,300 milligrams. Your body doesn't just use calcium to build bone; it relies on a steady supply for muscle contraction, to regulate blood pressure, and for healthy nerve function. What it doesn't get from your diet, it steals from your skeleton. Eat at least three servings of calcium-rich food—like skim milk, low-fat yogurt, and cottage cheese—a day.

Iron is essential for forming red blood cells, which, as you likely know, carry oxygen to your working muscles. Without enough iron, you get anemia, a fatiguing condition common among women, especially those of child-bearing age, many of whom not only don't eat enough iron-rich foods but also lose iron through menstruation each month. Good sources include seafood, fish, lean meat and poultry, nuts, fortified breads and cereals, and dark leafy green vegetables.

CAFFEINE

My favorite bike shop in the whole world is South Mountain Cycles & Coffee Bar in my hometown of Emmaus, Pennsylvania. I love it not just for its *Cheers*-like atmosphere where locals come and while away the hours but because it marries many riders' two true loves: coffee and cycling. Many a cyclist swears by starting each ride with a frothy cup of caffeine. With good reason.

A British review of twenty-one caffeine studies reported that the popular pick-me-up puts more pep in your pedaling while making tough efforts feel less painful. Exercisers who turbo charge with a pre-workout java jolt not only report lower ratings of perceived exertion but are able to ride significantly longer (and often faster) before tiring out. Australian researchers found that even a single cup of regular coffee drunk an hour before saddling up could increase cyclists' time to exhaustion by almost a third during a stationary bike test.

Why the dramatic benefits? For one, caffeine, as anyone knows, makes you more alert and attentive, so you're "up" for the task at hand. On the muscular level, it also stimulates the release and metabolism of fatty acids, which helps spare your precious glycogen stores. In one study, athletes who took about two cups of coffee's worth of caffeine before an exercise test boosted their circulating free fatty acids by 50%—a big benefit for regular riders who have become efficient fat burners.

A little Starbucks may also ease your pain. In one study in the aptly named *The Journal of Pain*, researchers found that cyclists who dosed on caffeine before a thirty-minute stationary bike test reported feeling substantially less muscle pain during their effort than those who pedaled caffeine-free. Another study from the University of Georgia found that women who took caffeine before a hard leg workout reported nearly half the amount of post-exercise soreness as their noncaffeinated counterparts.

One thing caffeine doesn't boost is your urine production. Long thought to be a diuretic, caffeine does not make you pee any more than equal amounts of noncaffeinated beverages, so it won't make you dehydrated.

Still, it's wise not to overdo it. Just 250 milligrams of caffeine—the amount in a tall Starbucks coffee—one to two hours before you ride does the trick. More can leave you jittery and anxious and can cause gastrointestinal distress. Of course, if you don't drink coffee or otherwise take in a lot of caffeine, this isn't a call to start. Some people are very sensitive to caffeine's stimulating effects. If you're one of them, it may cause more problems than performance benefits.

MEATLESS CYCLISTS

I grew up in a big hunting family. If it had fur, feathers, or fins, it graced our dinner table. Growing up, I had no moral objection. I still don't. But at some point shortly after high school, I decided I'd eaten my share of animals and stopped eating meat. I happily lived, trained, and raced that way for a dozen or so years. Though I've since become more flexitarian (I eat meat a few times a week) than vegetarian, I can attest that you can fuel your body just fine on plant foods.

Many sports nutritionists tell me they field more questions about vegetarianism than any other diet topic, likely because people still don't believe they can be competitive without being a carnivore. You most definitely can. For one, done right, vegetarianism is very healthy. Vegetarians tend to have lower body mass indexes, lower cholesterol rates, and lower cancer rates than people who eat a meat-centric diet. So their overall health skews better. Plus, because the average vegetarian consumes ample amounts of grains, beans, fruits, and vegetables, they're always carbo-loaded.

The performance problems veggie athletes run into center around protein. A diet of bagels, bananas, and pasta will not provide the complete arsenal of amino acids you need to repair the small tears and muscle damage that hard rides and workouts leave behind. Nor can it provide the protein needed for replenishing red blood cells and fortifying your immune system. The result can be constant soreness, fatigue, and vulnerability to every bug that makes the rounds. As mentioned, meat tends to supply complete proteins, while most plant foods (aside from soy) do not, so it's important to eat a well-rounded diet. Here are some tips for getting your protein fix:

GO FAUX

It's never been easier to eat vegetarian thanks to the astonishing array of "fake" meat foods available in every supermarket. Take your pick from veggie burgers, meatless sausages or ground beef or chicken, you name it, all 100% meat-free and made with soy protein.

ADD DAIRY

Eggs and milk serve up high-quality protein complete with all the amino acids you need. Unless you're a vegan (no animal-based foods of any kind, including butter and honey), these are ideal for fortifying a plant-based, vegetarian diet.

EAT TRADITIONAL ETHNIC DISHES

Mix and match veggie foods the right way and you make complete proteins. Borrow a page from traditional plant-based cuisines like Indian and Mexican food and mix grains with legumes. Beans and rice make a perfect protein.

EAT WHOLE FOODS

Because vegetarians sometimes miss out on minerals, including iron and zinc, that are abundant in meat, it's especially important they eat whole, unrefined foods like brown rice and whole wheat pasta, which have not been stripped of those minerals during processing. Also fill up on dark leafy greens, legumes, and dried fruit—all good mineral sources.

It's also important to eat enough food. It sounds funny to say that when most people are desperately trying to eat less. But the plant-based foods that compose a healthy vegetarian diet are relatively low in calories, fat, and protein, and high in fiber, which is bulky and slow to digest so you feel fuller faster. Eating more frequently—three meals and two snacks—throughout the day is one way to ensure adequate calories. Another is to add some calorie- and nutrient-dense foods into your diet. Nut butters, seeds, and oils help fuel you up as well as fill you up.

PAINLESS WEIGHT LOSS

Undoubtedly, many women use their bikes as a tool for weight loss (see page 119 for a "Weight Loss Plan"). And why not? Cycling is a great calorie burner. But there are a few common traps to watch out for. I know. When I first started racing, I actually gained weight. (I was recently reassured by the fact that I'm not the only one; a friend of mine just called to tell me she gained five pounds training for an Ironman triathlon). Here's how to avoid that same fate:

KNOW THE NUMBERS

You need to create a deficit of 3,500 calories to lose one pound. The best way to do that is exercise enough to burn an extra 250 (easily done through riding) and eat 250 fewer calories each day. That way you lose a pound a week. If you ride more or eat less, you'll lose a little faster, but most experts don't recommend losing more than two pounds a week, because that level of calorie deficit just isn't sustainable. Plus, you'll be hungry and cranky and have less energy to ride strong.

The only way to really know what you're burning and what you're eating is to do the math (the best you can—this isn't a perfect science) for a week. Recreational bicycling (12 MPH) burns about 450 calories an hour for a 140-pound woman. If you're lighter, you'll burn a little less; if you're heavier, you'll burn more. Now, read your labels and determine how many calories you're eating. At the end of the day, you should be eating fewer than you're riding off.

AVOID OVERCOMPENSATION

You just finished a two-hour ride and feel great. Still in your Lycra, you open the fridge and grab a glass of milk and a slice of cold pizza (hey, it's recovery, right?). You shower up and change and head out to run some errands. You stop at Starbucks. The cookies look so yummy, and, hell, you rode two hours today. Later at dinner, you have an extra glass of wine, because after all you rode two hours today . . . You get the picture (and this, by the way, was what caused my weight to creep for a short while). It's *very* easy to reward yourself all day for a ride you did at eight in the morning. If you burned 800 calories on your two-hour ride, you can afford to treat yourself to that recovery slice of pizza. But that's it for the day. Don't go overboard.

TIME YOUR NUTRIENTS

Riding off weight is easier if you think about food as fuel. Eat those tasty, bready carbs early in the day in the hours before you ride, when you need calories and carbs to energize you for the miles ahead. Have a skim mocha after your ride for a recovery boost. Then lighten your food intake as the day goes on and you become less active. Here is a sample of what a day in a cyclist's diet might look like:

- 7 A.M. Breakfast: 1 cup of cereal with 1/2 cup milk, piece of fruit, coffee or tea. Or two eggs with an English muffin and fruit.
- 10 A.M. Healthy snack (e.g., yogurt, fruit, nuts, fig bar)
- 12 P.M. Lunch: 1/2 turkey sandwich, 1 cup of soup, glass of milk, baby carrots. Or hummus wrap, mixed salad, milk.
- 3 P.M. Healthy snack (e.g., popcorn, nuts, small piece of dark chocolate, baby carrots)
- 6 P.M. Dinner: salmon steak, sautéed broccoli, brown rice, milk. Or chicken breast, roasted potatoes, asparagus, milk.
- 8:30 P.M. Healthy snack (same as above)

SAVOR EVERY BITE

Just as you should aim to enjoy every moment you're on the bike, try to savor every bite of food. Cycling allows you more freedom in what you eat; don't waste those earned calories by wolfing down your daughter's picked-over mac 'n' cheese or on some stale cookies that have been sitting in the office pantry for three days. Sit down and enjoy a great meal. Savor a small chunk of chocolate.

What you eat ultimately becomes part of your body, providing energy and immunity, and helps you live your life and ride your bike to the best of your potential. There's nothing else you put in your body so many times a day. Pay close attention to it, and you'll enjoy a robust riding career for years to come. *Bon Appétit!*

9

The Health of It

Fix What's Ailing You—Prevent What's Not

Thinking of driving to Canada to pick up some cheap prescription medicines? Ride your bike there instead. By the time you reach the border, you may not need them anymore. Riding a bike is such good medicine I've seen riders shed forty-plus pounds and tear up their Lipitor prescriptions after just a year of serious cycling.

RIDE YOUR WAY TO GOOD HEALTH

I'd go as far as to say that riding a bike will help you live longer. A recent study of more than 5,000 Americans found that people who participated in moderate exercise—and cycling's middle name is moderate—most of their lives collected about four more years at the end of the line.

Unlike running, which can be impossible for people with orthopedic issues, cycling is accessible to anyone with two decently functioning legs. (And, in fact, to those with just one. One of the regulars on our local Saturday morning shop ride has a prosthetic from the thigh down; you'd never know it from how he rides.) Start riding now, and there are a host of health problems you may be able to sail right by, or at least make a whole lot better.

LOWER HIGH CHOLESTEROL AND TRIGLYCERIDES

Cholesterol is an essential, waxy substance that drifts through your bloodstream along with other fats. Like Dr. Jekyll and Mr. Hyde, when it's good, it's very good (HDL—high-density lipoprotein—cholesterol, which sweeps excess fat from the blood), and when it's bad, it's really bad (LDL—low-density lipoprotein—cholesterol, which clogs up arteries). Triglycerides are another form of fat circulating through your system. Like cholesterol, a little is necessary, but too much is bad news. The American Heart Association recommends keeping total cholesterol below 240 (less than 200 is ideal), LDL under 130, and HDL above 40, though the higher the better. Triglycerides should be below 150 mg/DL.

Even a single bout of exercise can positively affect triglycerides. Riding enough to burn about 1,200 calories a week (that's just 30 minutes most days a week) can drop levels of these blood fats 25%. Riding improves cholesterol too, though some studies suggest it may take longer to make noticeable improvements. Higher intensity rides—those more than about 75% of your maximum heart rate range, or an 8 on a 1 to 10 exertion scale (see Chapter 5, "How to Train," for heart rate range and exertion guidance)—seem to be the ticket for really giving HDL a boost and for dumping dangerous LDL levels. Easy enough. Ride some hills or pedal hard into a headwind. A few hard efforts a week can help clean out your pipes and lower your risk.

DROP HIGH BLOOD PRESSURE

That beautiful beating heart of yours is happiest when your blood pressure (the pressure within your blood vessels as blood travels to and from your beating heart) is at 120/80 or lower. Higher than

140/90 and your risk for all kinds of dreadful health problems such as heart attack, stroke, and organ damage escalates.

The National Institutes of Health reports that aerobic exercise like cycling can reduce your systolic blood pressure (the top number) by an average of eleven points and your diastolic pressure (the bottom number) by an average of nine points. Research shows the best workouts for lowering blood pressure are the ones we all love best—long, steady spins that build our endurance and strengthen the cardiovascular system. Training three to five days a week at 65 to 70% of max heart rate—that's your comfortable aerobic zone, where you're breathing a little harder but could carry on a conversation—is ideal.

LOSE WEIGHT

Cute story: Last summer during a sixty-mile Sunday ride, three of my girlfriends and I stopped in a gas station to refill our water bottles (and grab a few doughnuts to refill our fuel tanks). As we were walking out, I heard the woman behind us in line say to her friend, "If riding a bicycle gives you a body like that, I'm gettin' me a bike!"

None of my friends nor I rides for weight control, but it sure is a nice fringe benefit of cycling. My friends span all ages from late twenties to mid-sixties, and they really do look amazing. At a time when most women are battling bulges, my forty-something friends can still button their blue jeans. They're not twigs. They're strong, healthy, vibrant (how many more positive adjectives can I use?) women who are really fun to go to dinner with because they never have to diet and always order dessert.

If your goal is to ride off your spare tire, do yourself a favor and forget all that hooey about "fat-burning zones." Yes, long easy rides through the country will burn plenty of calories, but to lose those love handles once and for all, you need to fire up your furnaces by pushing your body into the red once in a while. Jam up hills. Race your friends to street signs. Ride hard enough that you go "Whew!" when you're done. High-intensity efforts not only boost your calorie burn while you're riding; more important, your body needs more energy to recover, so you'll continue frying fat long after you're done.

Remember too that you gain innumerable health benefits even if you don't lose every last ounce you'd like. A growing body of evidence clearly shows that you can significantly lower your heart disease and diabetes risk by losing just 10% of your body weight. Ride your bike most days a week, and you'll lose that without even trying.

EASE ACHY JOINTS

Cyclists like to joke that eventually all runners find their way onto a bike. Cycling is gentle on the joints, and doctors consider it an excellent exercise option for people who have arthritis. Moving your joints maintains your range of motion and boosts circulation, so you transport nutrients into and metabolic waste out of the cartilage, keeping it healthier and helping prevent further degradation.

If you already suffer from chronic joint pain, it's important that you get in a good warm-up to really lubricate your joints before you turn up the intensity. In cycling specifically, try using lower gears and spinning faster to minimize any unnecessary torque in your hips and knees.

Fast pedaling drills are a fun way to increase your everyday riding cadence: Spin easy in a low gear for about 15 minutes. Gradually increase your cadence to 90 RPM. Hold there for 1 minute. Then increase to 100 RPM. Hold for 1 minute. Finally, take it to 110 and stay there for 5 minutes. Then bring it back down and finish your ride in a comfortable gear and cadence. Each ride try to increase the duration you spend at the fastest cadence, until you hit 15 to 20 minutes. Eventually a fast spin will feel like second nature.

GOOD FOR "GIRL" TROUBLES

Cycling is good for everybody. But it's especially good for the female body, because it tames out-of-control hormones and fends off female ills of all kinds. Here's what it can do for you.

Ease PMS

Back in the "good old days" menstruating women were often sent to the sidelines. Now we know that going out to play helps manage your periods. Studies show regular activity like cycling can help relieve that "I think I'll burn the house down today" tension as well as reduce cramping and general discomfort including headache and fatigue.

Some women worry that too much exercise may make them less fertile and therefore make it harder to have a baby when they want to get pregnant. Though it's true that intense training (e.g., high-volume triathlon training) may cause disruptions in your cycle, for the vast majority of women it's a nonissue. A survey of women training for the New York City Marathon showed that most had normal periods before and during their race training. The ones who didn't generally had a history of irregular periods before they started their marathon program. Usually women who develop amenorrhea (lose their periods) are also participating in sports that demand low body weight, so they are also dieting and often drop below a safe body-fat composition.

How well you perform during your period is another issue of hot debate, and research is all over the map as to whether you perform better or worse before, during, or after your period. So just listen to your body. If you feel miserable, take the day off, or go really easy and see if your symptoms subside. Technically speaking, it's probably best to wear a tampon when riding during your period. The chances of a pad staying put aren't great (though some light-day liners stay fairly secure), and wearing underwear with your cycling shorts increases the likelihood of uncomfortable chafing.

Help manage menopause

I am not yet going through menopause, so I'm going to take the word of those who are: It's not such an easy time. But moving your body helps . . . at least a little. Seriously. Your hormones have a profound effect on your mood, and during menopause your hormones are going through profound change. Riding your bike is not going to make all that go away. But it's a proven hormone helper.

Recently, Spanish researchers found that menopausal women who started a year-long exercise program enjoyed significant improvements in their mental and physical health, while those who stayed sedentary felt worse. The scientists asked forty-eight women ages fifty-five to seventy-two either to do some exercise for three hours a week or to go about their mostly sedentary lives as usual. At the start of the study, 50% of the women in the exercise group and 58% of the nonexercisers complained of severe menopause symptoms like fatigue and insomnia. By the study's end, the percentage of women with severe symptoms dropped to 37% among the active group and actually rose to 66% among the nonexercisers. The active women also reported better moods and mental well-being, while their couch-potato counterparts suffered a tougher time mentally and emotionally.

Again, cycling won't miraculously cool all those hot flashes (if only!), but it helps you sleep better, improves your mood, helps regulate your hormones, and puts your body in a healthier state at a time when other women are gaining weight and facing higher risks for heart disease.

Beat breast cancer

I've been following the research on prevention of breast cancer for an infuriating fifteen years. Broccoli prevents it. Well, no, it doesn't. Being overweight raises your risk. Well, maybe not. The Pill is safe. The Pill is dangerous.

The singular preventive measure that has stood the test of time, however, is exercise. Most recently, a twelve-year landmark study of 110,559 women reported that women who do vigorous exercise like spirited cycling five hours or more a week have a 20% lower risk of invasive breast cancer and a 31% lower risk of early stage breast cancer than their more sedentary peers. Another study of 15,000 women ages 20 to 69 reached a similar conclusion—that six hours of heart-pumping activity like brisk cycling a week can slash your risk of malignant breast cancer by 23%. Even better, the latter study found that the positive protection kicked in no matter when a woman jumped on the exercise wagon, so it's never too late to begin. What's more, riding your bike can also increase your likelihood of surviving breast cancer and can help smooth the road to recovery, according to a growing body of evidence.

Though scientists don't know exactly how exercise provides its breast protection, they suspect it works by lowering levels of female hormones like estradiol (a potent form of estrogen) and progesterone. However it works, it's another great reason to get on your bike as often as possible.

Lift depression

If I didn't ride my bike, I'd drink a lot more. And maybe I'd pick up the stupid smoking habit I dropped shortly after college. I, like many women (we suffer twice the rate of depression compared to men), have the specter of depression hovering around me almost constantly. The times it's blanketed me entirely are when I've been off my bike.

Exercise acts as an antidepressant, increasing the amount of serotonin that's available to the brain. Vigorous activity like cycling also boosts other feel-good chemicals, like endorphins—the opiatelike brain compounds that famously produce the "runner's high." For some, this cascade of positive effects works as well as medication against depression. In one study, men and women who worked out just thirty minutes a day three days a week reported the same relief from their depression symptoms as their peers who were on prescription meds. Even better, the exercisers were much less likely to have their symptoms return six months later.

Riding your bike will also make you more "stress resilient"—a jargony way of saying the more you ride, the more you'll be able to "go with the flow" in life without getting all bent out of shape. Scientists find that not only does regular activity help your body burn off harmful stress hormones; it also seems to train your central nervous system to better cope with such mental stresses as those from pressure-filled jobs and endless family obligations.

Escape bad relationships

Lousy relationships obviously aren't just a girl thing, but the women I know tend to hang around longer in bad situations than men do. Riding a bike gives them a vehicle to get out. Women who start cycling find joy. If you already have joy in your life, it's icing on the cake. If you don't, it's a revelation that you can actually feel so damn happy. Riding a bike also increases a woman's confidence. Riding a bike takes skill, fitness, and know-how. It's a reminder you have all that and more locked inside.

You'll also meet kindred spirits, which can help you find some really good relationships. Cycling's a really great way to meet and get to know someone. What else do you have to do to pass all those miles but talk? I'm not telling you to pick up a bike and dump that loser you're living with (unless you really are living with a loser). I've just seen countless women (like me!) and men find their way to happier lives and better bonds as a fringe benefit to this great sport.

But you need more for your bones

Cycling is one of the best exercises for every part of your body except the one that actually holds you together—your skeleton. One study has shown that voracious cyclists (those who are out spinning at least twelve hours a week) had bone densities 10% lower than their equally active, noncycling peers. This is especially concerning to women, especially those at risk for osteoporosis.

It's not that cycling is somehow inherently bad for your bones. It's just not all that good for them. Bones need impact to build, and as you likely know, cycling is a nonimpact sport, so it doesn't provide the right stimulus to build bone density. Mountain bikers fare a little better because they absorb some bumps and vibration from the rough terrain. But they too are wise to include some bone-building exercise in their regimen.

The easy answer is strength training, which all women should do anyway to prevent the muscle loss and metabolism meltdown that happens in our forties. Give your bones a much-needed boost twice a week with full-body strength training (for a full routine, see page 214). It doesn't take longer than fifteen or twenty minutes, and the improved muscle strength will also improve your riding.

PUTTING IT ALL IN PERSPECTIVE

Finally, don't beat yourself up if you've racked enough miles to make it to the moon and back and you still have bouts of the blues, suffer through crummy dinner dates, or need to pop pills to keep rising blood pressure in check. Like eating a healthy diet, riding your bike will undoubtedly help you be healthier, but some stuff is simply in the cards. I have a friend who rides like a pro and is built like a nymph, but hypertension is deep in her genes. She'll always need meds, but her daily rides help keep the rest of her health in check.

AVOIDING INJURY

Of course, if you're riding for your health, you want to keep your body free from the aches and pains that sometimes nag regular riders. Every sport has inherent risks. Cycling's biggest is obviously crashing. Though every rider hits the pavement at least once in their career, most often it's in a pretty unspectacular fashion, like falling over in the parking lot when trying to unclip from their pedals or skidding out on loose gravel. More common are muscle and joint pain that comes from poor bike fit or general overuse. Most of these can be avoided with proper fit (see page 37) and some simple preventive measures.

WEAR THE RIGHT STUFF

Cycling attire, specifically padded shorts and padded gloves, are designed to protect your "contact points" (the parts of your body that literally sit on the bike) from the wear and tear of absorbing road vibration and being in constant contact with the bike. Wear them every time you ride.

CHANGE HAND POSITION

Road handlebars provide myriad riding positions. You can put your hands in the drops, on the brake hoods, on the flat part of the bar tops. Each position puts pressure on a different part of your hand and also places your body in a slightly different riding position. Changing positions frequently will help keep your muscles fresh and will help prevent your hands from getting numb from all the pressure sitting in one place.

STAND UP ONCE IN A WHILE

Your butt gets tired sitting in a chair too long. It's no surprise that it might protest being perched on a bike saddle for hours without reprieve. Standing up once or twice an hour is like hitting "refresh." It gives your legs a quick stretch, takes the pressure off your posterior, and allows you to ride longer in greater comfort.

STAY LOOSE

Maintain a slight bend in your elbows and keep your upper body as relaxed as possible. Riding rigidly not only wastes energy; it places your muscles and joints at a higher risk for strains.

TROUBLESHOOTING: WHERE DOES IT HURT?

Even very cautious riders sometimes have aches and pains sneak up on them. When riders start increasing their miles, problems in bike fit or riding form that were previously unnoticeable become more pronounced. Below are some of the most common cycling woes and how to make them better (and stop them from happening again!):

SADDLE SORES

If you've ever sat on a fire ant (or a small colony of the "torch-erous" insects), you have a good idea what a saddle sore feels like. The worst ones I ever had were after a 40K bike leg of a triathlon in the pouring rain. I'd rubbed my soggy bum so raw that simply wearing pants hurt. "Saddle sore" is an umbrella term for any seat-induced pain in the butt. Most commonly, it's a chafed area that's been rubbed red from friction. It can also be an irritated hair follicle that turns into a painful pimplelike bump on your crotch or butt. They usually heal on their own if you show them some love and stay off your bike seat. But they can become infected if you're not careful, which leads to a festering mess. So it's better to catch them early or avoid them altogether.

The first line of defense is reducing friction. Lubricate the skin on your rear and crotch with a chamois cream, as described in Chapter 3, "Gearing Up." Dermatologists who ride often recommend A and D ointment for those prone to saddle sores because it contains vitamins A and D and zinc oxide to keep your skin healthy. Once you have a hot spot, help it heal quickly with a germ-killing antibiotic ointment like Neosporin.

While you're riding, make a conscious effort to move around on the saddle some. Women are generally more bottom heavy than men, and we have a tendency to park our behinds on the saddle and not move. Scoot forward, shift back, and stand up periodically to prevent one or two spots from taking all the pressure.

Once you're done with your ride, get out of your bike shorts ASAP (bacteria love to breed in warm, damp conditions) and shower up. If you can't hit the showers, at least wipe down your nether regions with a baby wipe.

NUMB HANDS OR FEET

Ever sleep on your arm funny and wake up with it numb? That's what happens to some riders when they put too much pressure on their hands and feet during long rides.

In the case of your hands, if they become numb when you ride, you're putting too much pressure on the palm of your hand and compressing either the median nerve (which runs through the carpal tunnel at the base of the hand and affects sensation of the thumb, first two fingers, and part of the ring finger) or the ulnar nerve (which goes through the Guyon's canal in the outer wrist and affects sensation in the pinkie and ring finger). If you feel like you're leaning heavily on your hands, chances are your bike fit isn't quite right. Go to your bike shop and have them check your bike position. Your hands should be perched comfortably on the bars with your wrists in a neutral (not excessively bent) position. You might need to raise your handlebar to achieve this. Padded cycling gloves also relieve pressure, as does cork handlebar tape.

Like numb hands, tingly toes and numb feet are also caused by too much pressure, either from above or below. Cycling shoes are made to fit snugly, but too often they're downright tight, cutting off circulation to your toes. Make sure you have plenty of room to wiggle your toes in your shoes. During long rides (especially in the summer) your feet may also swell. If your shoes start to feel uncomfortable, stop and loosen your straps.

Pressure on the balls of your feet also can cause problems by compressing the nerves that run to the front of your foot. You'll notice that cycling shoes aren't terribly well padded inside. If you're having foot pain or numb toes, try buying some insoles from the drugstore. They redistribute the pressure to a wider area of the foot.

BACK AND NECK ACHES

I don't know anyone whose back or neck hasn't protested at least a little during a very long ride. The reason why is obvious: You're bent forward for hours on end. Most of this garden-variety pain can be avoided and alleviated by changing riding positions frequently and consciously stretching out once in a while. Stand up on the pedals and press your hips forward to give your lower back a rest. Drop your head from side to side to relieve tired, tight neck muscles. If your aches and pains are persistent or show-stopping in intensity, there's likely a larger problem with your position or technique. Try the following:

Tweak your riding position

Proper bike fit works wonders for back and neck comfort. Pain in the neck and/or back usually indicates that you're too stretched out. Your stem may be too long, your saddle may be too far back, or your handlebar may be too low. Pain in the neck may also be a symptom of riding with handlebars that are too wide (women commonly have narrower shoulders than men). Swapping out your stem for one that is shorter (so you're less stretched out) and has more rise (brings your handlebars higher) often alleviates both of these problems. But the bottom line is you should take your bike to a professional at a bike shop for a better fit.

Train for the terrain

There are certain situations that will make your lower back cry uncle even on a perfectly fitting bike. Topping that list is long climbs. Your low back muscles support your trunk and provide a platform to push off of during seated climbs. As you climb more, you condition your lower back to withstand the stress. But if you've been riding and training on mostly flat to rolling roads and suddenly you take a long ride out into the mountains, you're bound to feel some backache. Give your back muscles time to adapt before you log a lot of mountainous miles. Also apply the advice on climbing in Chapter 4, "How to Ride" (see especially page 69). Easier climbing techniques such as downshifting and mixing standing with seated climbing can take a load of pressure off your lower back.

Strengthen your support system

As mentioned above, your back supports your upper body as you roll down the road. So do your abs, obliques, and the rest of your core, as the muscles that surround your torso have become popularly known. Though cyclists rely heavily on their core to stabilize themselves in the saddle and put power in their pedals, cycling does very little to strengthen this important support system. All riders—even if they've never had the slightest twinge of back pain—should work on strengthening their back and abs. For specific exercises, see Chapter 5, "How to Train" (p. 91).

Limber up your limiters

Tight hamstrings and hips can make it impossible to position your pelvis in a neutral position—not tilted too far forward or back—on your saddle. Any pulling or compressing can cause pain in your back. The cycling-specific flexibility stretches found on page 220 can keep those hips and legs loose so they aren't constantly stressing your back.

KNEE PAIN

Bicycling is often prescribed for rehab after knee surgery because it's so gentle on the joints. Yet, ironically, knee pain is one of the leading ailments that stop recreational cyclists in their tracks. It's really a matter of math. If you turn your pedals at the suggested 90 revolutions per minute, that means you're cranking out 5,400 pedal strokes an hour—27,000 a week if you take a short ride most days. That means any little thing that tweaks your knee—be it poor bike position or pedaling technique—gets multiplied literally tens of thousands of times.

At the risk of sounding like a broken record, make sure your bike fits properly. Being too far forward, back, up, or down can impact your knees' well-being. As a rule of thumb, if your knees are starting to hurt in the back, lower your saddle a touch. If they're hurting in front or the sides, raise the saddle. If that doesn't work, get a professional fit.

Next, check your cleats if you ride clipless pedals. Misaligned cleats are a major source of knee problems. Your cleats should be positioned so that the ball of your foot is directly over the axle of the pedal. They should also be aligned so your toes point forward in a neutral position, not out or in, when you're on the bike. Most cleat/pedal systems today have "float," which means your feet are not locked solid in one position, and you can swivel your foot around a little bit without disengaging the cleat from the pedal. For knee health, most sports med experts recommend that your pedals have about 5 to 6 degrees of float. (Most pedals provide this information in their packaging.)

I've had my bike professionally fit and my cleats aligned, yet come spring, I often end up with a minor bout of knee pain. Why? Overzealousness. I get swept up in the sunny weather and go out and ride some stupid distance before I've properly trained. Fortunately, it's generally not something a little Advil and ice can't help. But knee pain can be chronic so it's best to play it smart and avoid doing too much too soon—the most common source of early season knee pain. Ramp up your mileage gradually, increasing your total weekly saddle time by no more than about 10% a week.

Cozy knees are healthy knees, as the blood and synovial (joint lubricating) fluids flow easily. Cover your hinges with knee warmers, tights, or knickers when the temps dip below 65 degrees. Warm up your knees from the inside out as well. Always warm up for a good ten minutes of easy spinning before you start riding hard.

Finally, save the mashing for your potatoes. Even if your legs are strong enough to push a huge gear, your knees likely aren't strong enough to withstand the shearing force. Remember to keep your cadence on the higher side, especially when climbing. When your cadence starts to dip, either downshift or get out of the saddle to take the pressure off your knees.

VAGINA WOES

If my vagina did a monologue during my last 500-mile bike tour, it would have sounded something like: "[Bleep]! Why? [Bleep]! Not again! [Bleep]!" I wore some old (but very cute) shorts the first 118-mile day and, well, that didn't go over so well down below. Women have this little problem that our insides (the tender tissues of our vagina) are sitting precariously close to our outsides (the vulva that perches on the saddle). Usually this isn't a problem, but once you aggravate those tender tissues, they pipe up pretty loudly.

High-quality, women-specific cycling shorts that have a molded, one-piece padded liner without irritating seams will baby your tender tissues on even the roughest rides. With age, our labia also lose a little bit of padding. If padded shorts aren't providing enough protection, seek out a women-specific saddle as well. They're anatomically designed to support your wider pelvis and often have cutouts in the nose to relieve pressure. This may be hard to believe, but the right saddle is as comfortable as an easy chair (truly). So keep trying until you get one that, in the immortal words of Goldilocks, feels "just right."

Some women also find that their occurrence of bladder infections increases with their miles logged. That's because anything that irritates your urethra increases the risk of bacteria sneaking into the bladder and setting up a colony. The right shorts and saddle should eliminate this problem. For extra insurance, reduce the concentration of bacteria in your bladder by drinking plenty of fluids on the bike (a bottle an hour) and peeing when you need to.

THE SHAPE OF YOUR LIFE

Our local cycling clubs are filled with riders in their fifties, sixties, and beyond. And that's one of the things I like best about the sport. It's something you can do for the rest of your life. Take care of your body with a good bike fit and smart cycling routine, and you can enjoy the sport for decades to come.

10

Get Your Hands Dirty

A Little Basic Bike Maintenance and Repair Is a Must

Honestly, I feel a little hypocritical writing this chapter. I love riding bikes. I love looking at bikes. I love writing about bikes. I'm not so hot on cleaning, maintaining, and working on bikes. When I get a flat on a group ride, I silently jump for joy when someone (usually a guy . . . hey, I'm not above accepting chivalry) steps up and offers to fix it. But when I'm out there by myself, I'm "the guy" who has to make simple repairs. I've also put a few dents in my MasterCard replacing pricey components that would have lasted longer if I'd just practiced some basic maintenance.

That's a long way of saying that even if you've got a standing appointment with your manicurist, you're going to need to get your hands a little greasy once in a while. There are entire, big fat books written about bicycle maintenance and repair (*Bicycling Magazine's Complete Guide to Bicycle Maintenance and Repair for Road and Mountain Bikes* is a classic), and I'm not a mechanic, so I'm not going to go into painstaking detail about changing brake pads or fixing your bottom bracket—leave that to the shop. Let's just focus on the simple stuff that will help your bike run better longer and will prevent you from hoofing it home or calling for a ride when you run into a little trouble on the road or trail.

A FEW SIMPLE REPAIRS

Most bikes run amazingly well with very little mechanical trouble. But flat tires happen to everyone sometime. And, over time, bolts can come a little loose, especially on mountain bikes. Here's how to manage these most basic repairs. You can learn more about bike mechanics by taking a class through your bike shop or buying a manual as mentioned above.

FIXING A FLAT

Even if you learn no other repairs, learn this one. Ride long enough and you will get a flat. They don't happen often; I've gone years without any. But there's no way to ride without fixing a flat when it does happen. Here's a step-by-step guide:

Remove the wheel

The first step to fixing a flat is getting the wheel off the bike. If the flat is in the back, shift into the smallest chainring and rear cog (this creates some slack in the chain and makes removing the wheel easier).

Then open the brakes. On road bikes, you'll see a little lever on the side of the braking mechanism. Lift that up, and you'll see the brake pads open wide, making room for your tire to pass through. If you don't see a lever, look for a button on the brake levers on the handlebars and push that button. Mountain bikes often have linear or V-pull brakes. Release those by squeezing the braking mechanism and lifting the brake cable out of its holder. Cyclocross bikes have cantilever brakes with a cable running on top of the tire; open those by releasing the cable from its holder near the brake pad on either side of the wheel. Disc brakes require no special steps; the disc simply slides out of the braking mechanism. This all sounds much more complicated than it is. When you look at the braking mechanism, it will be apparent where the brakes release.

Next, open the quick release. Your wheel stays attached to the bike frame (the hooks that hold them are called the "dropouts") via a skewer with a locking mechanism known as a "quick release." Open the lever (it should be firmly cinched down) and hold the lever in place while turning the cap on the other side of the wheel a few times to loosen the release enough to remove the wheel.

Finally, remove the wheel. Front wheels are a breeze to take off. Rear wheels require more finagling. Pull the derailleur back and hold it there, so it and the chain are out of the way as you remove the wheel. Once the wheel is off, lean the bike over on its left side, so you don't get your chain all dirty while you fix the flat.

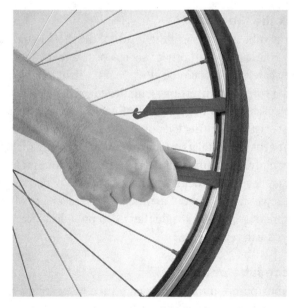

Tire levers make it easier to remove the tire and remove the punctured tube.

Release the tire and remove the tube

Time to pull out your tire levers, spare tube, and pump (see "Fix-it Kit," page 44) and get to work.

If the tire is not already completely flat, fully deflate it. For Presta valves, unscrew the top and press down to let the air out. For Schrader valves, stick an end of your tire lever into the valve and press the tip to release the remaining air. For Presta valves, once the air is out, remove the nut at the base of the valve to allow the tube to be removed.

Lever time. Hold the wheel up so the valve is at the bottom and wriggle a lever between the rim and the tire and wedge it underneath the edge (called the "bead") of the tire. Pry the tire off the rim and hook the lever to a nearby spoke. Now take another lever and do the same thing several inches away from the first lever. Repeat with the final lever. At this point, you should be able to remove that entire side of the tire out of the rim and pull out the tube. (If not, remove the first lever and pry off another spot until the tire comes loose.)

Check the tire

Once the tube is out, check the inside of the tire for sharp objects. Sometimes you can see a thorn or sharp rock. Other times you may have to very carefully (it could be glass, so use a light touch so as not to cut yourself) run your fingertips along the edges. It's possible that the offending item fell out when you pulled out the tube or that it punctured the tire without getting lodged inside. But it's important to check so you don't get a second flat immediately after changing the first.

Occasionally, you'll find a large gash or worn spot in the tire. This makes it easy for sharp rocks and rough road to penetrate and pop your tube. To get home without another flat, place a piece of duct tape or a dollar bill over the area inside the tire to provide a layer of protection until you can replace the tire.

Replace tube and tire

With your pump, inflate your spare tube just enough so it takes shape. Holding the wheel upright with the valve hole at the top, place the valve into the hole and tuck the tube into the tire and onto the rim, with both hands, working your way down to the bottom of the wheel.

Now work the tire back onto the rim (this can be the hardest part). Starting at the valve, work the tire bead back into the rim using the palms of your hands. You can also use your lever to push it back into place. When you get to the bottom, it will become more difficult. Be sure that the valve is fully through the hole. If it feels impossibly tight, remove some air from the tire. Then wriggle the final few inches of the tire back on the rim.

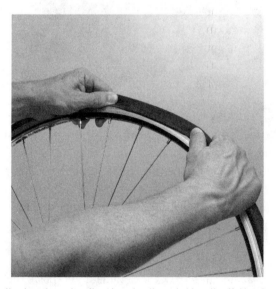

Putting the tire back on is often harder than taking it off. Use two hands to work it back into place.

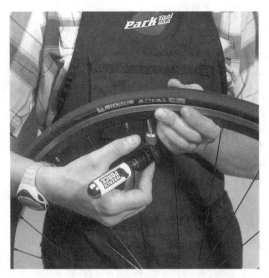

A CO_2 cartridge makes inflating tires a breeze!

Reinflate, "reverse," and roll

Once the tire is back in place, add a little air and check that the tire is seated correctly on the rim. Look between the rim and the tire to be sure the tube isn't sticking out anyplace (if the tube gets trapped under an edge, it can pop). Then finish inflating the tire. If you're using a mini-pump, you may not be able to get it 100% firm; just top it off with your floor pump when you get home.

Then put the tire back on, reversing the steps you did to take it off. For the rear tire, pull back the derailleur and place the chain over the smallest cog (where it was when you removed it). Then wiggle the skewer back into the dropouts. Tighten the quick release until you feel some resistance, then close it so the lever points up and aligns with the fork. It should be tight enough that it takes firm pressure to close the lever but not so tight that you can't fully close it. Close the brakes or reattach the brake cable, and you're ready to roll.

If you've never fixed a flat, practice at home, so you feel confident in your ability out on the road or trail. The first time, it may take you twenty minutes to figure it all out. But once you get the hang of it, it's a very quick repair.

PATCHING A TUBE

Just as you can go years without getting a flat, you can inexplicably get two in one day. When that happens, you can just patch the tear and keep on rolling. To patch a tube, you first need to find the hole. With larger tears, it can be obvious just by looking. Smaller holes can be tough to see. If you can't find it, inflate the tire and put it up to your ear, rotating it around until you hear the hissing of leaking air. Then inspect that area closely until you find the hole.

Follow the directions on the patch kit to repair the hole. Generally, with regular patches, you scuff the tire around the hole with a little sandpaper (provided in the kit), then apply a thin layer of glue, let the glue dry a little, and press on the patch. Then the tire is as good as new.

TIGHTENING LOOSE BOLTS

It's a good idea to periodically check the bolts on your bike, particularly those on your handlebars, cranks, chainrings, water bottle cages, and seat post for tightness. But let's face it, that's easy to forget, so you may find yourself out on the road with a rattling, loose bottle cage or a seat that keeps sliding down. Easy fixes.

Take out your multi-tool or Allen wrenches and simply cinch them down. Turn the wrench just until the bolt is firmly in place; don't crank it down with all your might. That's how bolts break.

BASIC BIKE CARE

Again, I'm far from meticulous about bike maintenance. But after having to replace expensive components that would have lasted longer had I just cleaned and lubed them once in a while, I've learned that a little love goes a long way in keeping your bike running smoothly. Here are the basic bike care essentials you need to know:

PUMP YOUR TIRES

Properly inflated tires are less prone to flats, ride more smoothly, and protect your bike's rims from getting beat up and bent. Even if you never puncture your tubes, your tires eventually will go flat because air seeps out of the relatively porous rubber. Make it a habit to pump your tires before every ride, if possible, or at least once a week.

Road bike tires take considerably more pressure (pounds per square inch, or PSI) than mountain bike tires. Check the tire's sidewalls for the manufacturer's recommended pressure and keep your tires inflated to that level.

LUBE YOUR CHAIN

Just as motor oil keeps your engine from seizing up, bike lube keeps your chain and gears from grinding together and wrecking your drivetrain (I've had to replace my gears prematurely because I neglected to keep my chain lubed). The most important part to keep lubricated is your chain. A well-lubed chain shifts and runs more smoothly than a dry one.

To lube your chain, turn the bike upside down (or hang it from a stand or hook) and apply one drop of lube to each link as you slowly pedal backward. Once you've gone all the way around, continue pedaling for a few seconds to let the lube work its way into the chain. Then take a rag and gently press it against the chain as you pedal backward to wipe off the excess lube (the lube is meant to be in your chain, not coating the outside, collecting grime). If you're using one of the self-cleaning lubes, you may need to apply a little more to saturate the chain, so it can dissolve the gunk. Just follow the directions on the package.

It's a good idea to lube your chain after every few rides, about once a week or so, and always after riding in the rain, since water washes away the lube.

CHOICES, CHOICES

The bike lube market is as saturated as a McDonald's french fry. There are lubes made from oil, silicone, wax, and a combination of ingredients. There are self-cleaning lubes (which means you don't wash the chain before applying), lubes you spray on, and lubes you drip on. Which you choose depends on the conditions in which you ride as well as personal preference.

Generally speaking, you can divide lubes into three categories: dry, wet, and wax.

Dry lubes: These go on wet but then set up mostly dry. They often contain synthetics like Teflon, and they run smoothly and hold up well. For many riders, dry lubes are ideal because they don't attract or absorb much dirt, making them good for dusty or off-road conditions.

Wet lubes: These liquid lubes go on wet and stay wet. They stand up to rainy, wet weather. They do attract grime, and you have to clean your chain a little more often. Wet lubes are very durable, so if you ride the road and in mostly clean conditions, these are a good choice.

Wax lubes: As the name implies, these lubes dry to a hard wax. Their big advantage is they don't attract dirt or dust, so they keep your chain clean. They're very popular among mountain bikers for that reason. The downside is they're not very durable, and you have to relube often—every other ride or so.

Self-cleaning lubes: These are wet-style lubes that not only hold up well in wet-rainy conditions but work to lift the old lube and grime out from the chain and leave behind a clean coat. No separate cleaning required.

Other parts that might need lubing include your cleats and/or pedals if you're using a clipless pedal system, the pivots around your derailleur and brakes, and any spinning parts that contain bearings. Follow the instructions that come with your shoes/pedals, and once a year take your bike to the shop for a full lube job. Late winter, early spring is the perfect time, since your bike has likely sat unused for a few weeks (or maybe even months) and could use a tune-up anyway. Don't wait too long to bring your bike in. Bike shops get *really* busy when the weather gets nice. Aim for late February or early March.

CHECK YOUR BRAKES

For obvious reasons, it's important to keep this part of your bike well maintained. Keep your rims and brake pads free from debris (this is especially true if you're riding off-road or in wet conditions where lots of dirt and grime kick up and get stuck on these components). If you see black streaks (rubber deposits from the brakes) on your rims, wipe them off with a rag dipped in a little rubbing alcohol. Give your brake pads a wipe while you're at it, especially if you see rubber shreds or road dirt on them.

Every time you squeeze your brakes, they wear down a tiny bit. It's important you don't let them wear all the way down, or you'll be rubbing metal on metal (the brake pad holder on the rim), which not only doesn't stop you very well but wrecks your rims. Take a look at your brake pads every once in a while. New pads have grooves to help channel water away from the rims and allow the brakes to get a better grip in wet conditions. When those grooves become faint, it's time to replace the pads. Your bike shop can do it in a snap.

CLEAN IT UP

A clean bike is a happy, well-running bike. All you need is a hose, a bucket, and a few sponges and/or brushes. When your bike is dirty with road grime or muddy from riding on the trail, take it out in the yard and hose it down. Resist the temptation to blast away at the drivetrain or moving parts with a strong stream of water, because you can end up with water in your bottom bracket and other places you don't want it. Instead, gently spray it from above, taking care not to hit the lubed parts (e.g., the chain) with too much force.

Once you've showered off the worst of the crud, fill the bucket with soapy water (dish detergent works well) and scrub it down, using a small sponge or brush to clean all the nooks and crannies. Wipe the bike dry with a clean towel, relube the chain, and you're good to go.

You can make this job even easier with a special bike cleaning kit that includes a variety of brushes and cleaning fluids specially designed to reach and clean all your bike's hard-to-clean parts, like around the brakes and gears. You'll find them at your local bike shop.

KEEP IT SAFE

Your bike will last longer and look better if you store it inside, away from the elements. Many cyclists hang their rides on bike hooks in the garage, mudroom, or rec room. These are rubber-covered sturdy hooks that screw into the ceiling or wall (be sure you secure it in a beam or stud, so the bike doesn't fall) that you hook through one of your bike wheels to hang it out of harm's way, where it won't get knocked over or scratched by items leaning or falling against it.

Another option is a bike stand, similar to what mechanics use in bike shops. These stands hold the bike with a clamp that closes around the seat post. Like hooks, they get the bike up off the floor and away from traffic. They're also very functional, providing a place to hang your bike at eye level, so you can lube your chain, check your brakes, and make small repairs or adjustments.

LOOK IT OVER

A good bike frame can last you a lifetime. But components like tires, cables, hubs, and bottom brackets don't last forever. Inspect your bike once a month or so. Look for frayed cables, worn tires, torn handlebar tape, loose bolts on your chainrings, rust spots, and cracks in the plastic housing that surrounds your cables by the shifters and brakes. If you see anything that looks worn out, broken, or not quite right, take it to your shop for an evaluation and possible repair or replacement.

While you're at it, give the bike frame, fork, and handlebars a once-over. Depending on your bike materials and the terrain or road conditions you typically ride, it's not impossible to crack your fork, handlebars, or even frame, which as you can imagine is potentially disastrous. This is a rare occurrence, of course, but it is always smart to err on the side of safety.

A LITTLE TLC GOES A LONG WAY

For some people, bike care becomes a hobby. They get great pleasure out of fine-tuning, tweaking, cleaning, and tinkering with their bikes. You don't have to be one of those people to keep your bike riding its best. Simply keeping it clean and well cared for, fixing things as they break, and repairing parts as they wear will guarantee you miles of enjoyment for many years to come.

11

Time to Ride

Becoming a Cyclist Takes More Than Intent

 If you're one of those lucky women who "have it all"—the job, the family, the house, or some combination of the above—there's probably just one thing in your life that's missing: time!

Even women who really love cycling often struggle to carve out an hour (or on good days more) to ride amidst all the demands of commuting, career, and caretaking. Women, more than men, also have a tendency to feel guilty about taking time away from social obligations and the daily to-dos to break free for some simple playtime. But it can—and should—be done. The women I know who make it work—and, yes, that includes women with full-time jobs and full houses of three (or more!) kids—do so by making riding a priority. Like anything that's important to them, they're willing to leap some hurdles to make it happen.

THE RIGHT TIME

First, toss out the words "I don't have time." Busy is the new normal, and it's no longer a good excuse for neglecting your needs. The key is finding time you didn't know you had and using the time you do have more wisely. Here's how:

RISE AND RIDE

This is my personal favorite and a tip that topped the list when I asked my cycling buddies how they squeeze more rides into the week. Life starts pitching surprises as the day wears on, and by five thirty p.m. you can almost guarantee you'll get hit with a curveball that threatens to waylay your riding plans. By getting out the door early, you avoid those distractions. As a bonus, you also avoid a lot of traffic and, in the summer, the scorching heat of the day. By the time you get to work, your workout is done, and the day is yours. All these benefits may be why research consistently shows that morning exercisers stick to their routines better than those who try to fit it in at other times of the day.

Of course, this means leaving your soft, warm bed earlier than usual, and that is *anything* but easy. I'm a morning person and an avid cyclist, and I still wrestle the urge to roll over and get more *zzz*s when the alarm goes off. Make it hard to talk yourself out of riding by placing all your clothes in a neat pile directly in your line of sight from the pillow before you go to bed. Also prepare your water bottles and have them in the fridge ready to go. If you go to the trouble to pave the way the night before, you'll be far less likely to let yourself down come morning.

TAKE A POWER LUNCH

There's a group of cyclists in my town who meet at high noon every day year-round to ride on their lunch hour. This is an excellent option if you can swing it. It takes a little preparation. You have to find a place to ride. Local parks are a great option if you're in the city. Or maybe you can find some back roads to string together a ten- or fifteen-mile loop if you work in a more suburban or rural setting. You also need to pack your stuff and be a quick-change artist in the office restroom. But once you try it, you'll be hooked. This midday "brain shower"—as a friend of mine calls it—improves your mood, refreshes your energy, and boosts your productivity for the rest of the day. Then you can just grab a healthy lunch (or bring one with you) to eat at your desk when you're done.

Two questions that inevitably come up when cyclists talk about lunch rides is showering and helmet hair. If your office building has a shower facility and locker room (many do), you're in luck. But, truthfully, you don't necessarily need a shower, even after a sweaty ride. Baby wipes or products like Rocket Shower spray body cleaner will leave you feeling fresh in a snap. As for your hair, a little gel or mousse and a blast with a hair dryer (pack a mini one in your duffle bag) will help lift it back in place.

USE THE EVENING HOURS

Post-work is undoubtedly one of the most popular times to work out—just try to get on any gym treadmill at six p.m. But it's also a popular time for baseball practice, scout gatherings, school board meetings, and a host of other extracurricular and community activities. Your best bet is to schedule your evening rides as you would any other meeting. Put it on the calendar and commit to it. And get creative. You don't really have to stand there (or sit in your car) during Emily's dance class or soccer scrimmage. Throw your bike in the car and use her practice time to get some exercise of your own.

COMMUTE

Before people rode bikes for exercise and fun, they rode them as transportation. More than half of Americans live less than five miles from where they work, and, in light of rising fuel costs and global climate changes, many are discovering that getting there by bike saves money and emissions with a side benefit of getting in shape.

Depending on your commute, you may ride your bike on the same roads you typically drive your car. Or you may need to choose a path that avoids interstates or otherwise unsafe roads. Your bike shop may have maps that show cycling-friendly roads in your region so you can try different routes. Another option is visiting www.mapquest.com. Choose driving directions from your street address to your work address, then click "Advanced Options" and "Avoid Highways." The directions that pop up should provide the shortest route using back roads.

Generally speaking, commuting by bike will take about twice as long as driving, unless you live within seven miles of your job. Then it may be even faster (this has been my experience). A study by New York City's Transportation Alternatives shows that trips of less than three miles are often faster by bike, and those five to seven miles in length take about the same time. How can that be? Because as a cyclist riding on the shoulder, you can pass long lines of traffic crawling along clogged streets.

Even if it does take longer, spending an extra thirty minutes getting to work is the beauty of bicycle commuting. When the day is done, you've racked up an hour of riding without having to make time to get on your bike. It's an easy way to get lots of exercise during the hectic workweek. And it counts as training if you're preparing for an event.

Can't commit to a long commute? Slice it down to size. Many bus and rail lines allow cyclists to bring their bikes on board (you may need a permit, so check in advance), so you can ride your bike to a designated park-and-ride lot and catch a train or bus the rest of the way. Or drive halfway to work and leave your car at a shopping center or safe place to park, then ride your bike the rest of the way.

A roomy backpack or bike messenger bag makes it easy to carry your clothes and work-related items. Or, if you're worried about wrinkly pants, you can just bring extra outfits to work on the days you drive. Even if you commute by bicycle just one or two days a week, you've gotten in miles you otherwise would have missed, and you've done your share to help keep our planet healthy.

USE THE WEEKENDS WISELY

Saturday and Sunday mornings (or late afternoons) are perfect for long, rambling rides. Get up early and you can sail around for two blissful hours and still get back in time to have breakfast with the family. Even if you have other obligations, you can usually squeeze in a ride around them. Friends of mine ride to their kids' soccer games (of course, one parent has to be available to drive the kids there), and I've even been known to ride to church.

To get better at cycling, it helps to ride at least three or four days a week. The weekend is your chance to seize two days without the time constraints of work.

LET THE SMALL STUFF SIT

If you become an avid cyclist, you will probably not have an immaculate house. Make peace with it and move on. For some women, this is the highest hurdle in finding time to ride. There's the dishes and the laundry and the stacks of mail on the table and the litter box. Well, those messes are constant. More important, they can wait until the sun goes down. Your ride can't.

One of my favorite tricks is to include "ride" on my daily to-do list or weekend agenda. It prioritizes it right up there with "groceries" and "weed flowerbed," and I feel just as satisfied when I get to check it off the list as accomplished.

IT'S A FAMILY AFFAIR

Time to ride doesn't have to be time away from your family if you take them with you. One of my best friends, Christine, is a mom of two young boys and the wife of a chef who travels a lot. Sometimes she hires a babysitter so she can get out for long rides. But often she just takes the kids with her, in bike seats and toddler trailers when they were little and now that they're older on bikes of their own.

"I've ridden with them at the park and on the road. I've done hill repeat workouts pulling them in a trailer. You name it," she says.

Another friend makes it a point to do the MS 150 (a 2-day, 150-mile charity ride) with his family every summer, so they train together. Other friends set up their indoor trainer in the living room and ride while watching a movie with their too-young-to-ride kids. My daughter's favorite activity is riding on the Trail-a-Bike (a little "half bike" that attaches to the back of your bike) around our neighborhood. It may not be training as I traditionally think of it. But it sure is exercise!

If your family isn't into cycling, consider other options. You can ride while the kids go in-line skating. You can ride while your husband jogs. Or pull a swing shift. Maybe your husband golfs or has another hobby. Take turns. You ride in the morning, he plays nine holes in the afternoon, and you reconvene for dinner in the evening. Active couples who both ride also find that it works to befriend other cycling couples. Then they trade kid-sitting detail, so each couple can actually get out and ride together.

What if no one is active but you? And worse, they resent your riding time? One word: communication. Your partner is not a mind reader. Nor are your kids. If they expect you to be around Saturday morning, it's not surprising that they'll feel disappointed when you spring it on them that you're off for a two-hour ride. Let them know your plans, so they can figure them into their own. Without climbing onto any tall horses or soapboxes, communicate with your family that riding is important to you and the time you spend on your bike makes you a happier mom and companion when you're home.

KEEP ON KEEPING ON

I love cycling, yet I still have days when it's a struggle to hoist myself out of my chair and saddle up for a ride. Motivation is the same for all of us: It waxes and wanes like the moon. You just need a few little tricks to keep yours shining bright when it would otherwise dim. Here are a few favorites:

FIND A FRIEND . . . OR FOUR

Remember how as a kid you'd bang on every door on the block or call every friend in a five-mile radius until you found someone to come out and play? When you did, you'd tear up the neighborhood until your mom called you for dinner. And if you didn't? You'd mope back home and veg in front of the TV. You may be bigger now, but you're likely still a kid at heart, and it's still more fun to play with friends.

If none of your friends ride, it's easy enough to find some who do. Head to your local bike shop and ask around. Start going on organized group rides. Join a bike club. Once you hook into the cycling circle in your area, you'll find plenty of like-minded people to play with.

SIGN UP FOR SOMETHING

Nothing gets you out on your bike like knowing you have a 100-mile ride to do in five weeks. Signing up for a bike tour vacation or a big single-day ride will give you all the more reason to get up and go when you feel like staying put. Local bike clubs are great sources of information on races, rides, and organized cycling events throughout the year.

DO IT FOR CHARITY

Name the cause and there's likely a ride for it. I've pedaled to raise money for AIDS vaccines, multiple sclerosis research, diabetes funds, heart disease organizations, terminally ill children, and to help find a cure for cancer. Riding for worthy causes reminds you that it's a privilege to have a healthy, able body to ride a bike and fuels your motivation because you know you're doing good for more than yourself. Web sites such as www.active.com can help you find charity events in your area.

LIE TO YOURSELF

When you're feeling really lazy, sometimes it helps to fib to yourself. Tell yourself that you'll just go out and spin easy for twenty minutes just to do *something*. Once you're out there, there's no way you're turning back in twenty (and deep inside you know that). But giving yourself permission to bail if you're not having fun is often all you need to get rolling in the right direction.

JUST DO IT

Above all, enjoy the sport. Don't be hard on yourself if you miss a few days or your big local hill still gets the best of you. Don't sweat it if your bike isn't as fancy as everyone else's or you haven't quite got the hang of clipless pedals.

Your cycling will evolve with your life. Some seasons everything will just click. You'll feel super fit and be riding all the time. Other seasons, life will get in your way and slow you down. Just keep putting one pedal in front of the other and enjoy the ride and all the rewards it has to offer.

Index